Homemade
HERBAL
MEDICINE

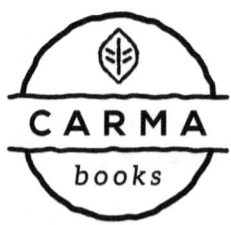

'A conscious approach to health & wellness'

carmabooks.com

*You are invited to to join our **Free Book Club** mailing list. Sign up via our website to receive **special offers** and **free for a limited time** Health & Wellness eBooks!*

Homemade
HERBAL
MEDICINE

Your Essential Guide to Herbs & DIY Remedies for Health & Healing

Carmen Reeves

Disclaimer

This book provides general information and extensive research regarding health and related subjects. The information provided in this book, and in any linked materials is for informational purposes only, and is not intended to be construed as medical advice. Speak with your physician or other healthcare professional before taking any nutritional or herbal supplements. There are no 'typical' results from the information provided - as individuals differ, the results will differ. Before considering any guidance from this book, please ensure you do not have any underlying health conditions which may interfere with the suggested healing methods. If the reader or any other person has a medical concern or pre-existing condition, he or she should consult with an appropriately licensed physician or healthcare professional. Never disregard professional medical advice or delay in seeking it because of something you have read in this book or in any linked materials. The reader assumes the risk and full responsibility for all actions, and the author or publisher will not be held liable for any loss or damage that may result from the information presented in this publication.

Carma Books
carmabooks.com

hello@carmabooks.com

CONTENTS

CHAPTER 2

CHAPTER 3

CHAPTER 4

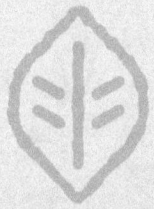

INTRODUCTION

I want to thank you for your recent purchase of my latest piece on health and wellness: *Homemade Herbal Medicine, Your Essential Guide to Herbs & DIY Remedies for Health and Healing.*

If you are a passionate follower of my other Carma Books publications, you have probably noticed well by now how important I deem the use of plants and botanical medicine in holistic healing. Herbs are miraculous saviors for such an extensive list of issues you can handle at home: gut health, inflammation, and even health maladies as complex as thyroid issues and adrenal fatigue.

But do herbs really work? Can they really help you feel empowered, and take control over at least some of your health? Maybe those questions led you to obtaining this book. Or maybe, like me, you already love herbs so much that you can't hold back from buying any literature you find!

My immediate answer to these questions? **Yes!** I've studied and apprenticed for many years as a lover and huge "herb nerd," and I've seen how the use of herbal remedies can slowly, subtly, and powerfully change peoples' lives. Even better—there is plenty of research supporting herbs for personal care, too.

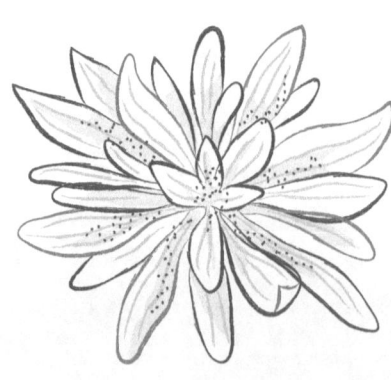

If you get to know and use herbs correctly, you can see those very same changes in your own life—sometimes, in ways you never thought imaginable. Rest assured, this book will show you how.

What is Herbal Medicine?

Herbal medicine, also called "herbalism" or sometimes "herbology," is the ancient practice of using the plants around us—in nature, or our gardens—to promote healing.

Long before modern medicine and the techniques of surgery, technology, pharmaceuticals and vaccines, people all around the world depended on herbs to protect their health and ward off even the gravest of illnesses.

Depending on the culture, country, or region, there are hundreds of traditions of herbal practice that existed long before the advent of modern-day techniques. In fact, while "conventional medicine" may seem like the more dominant form of healing, **statistically speaking the World Health Organization marks traditional medicine (including herbalism) the most prevalent form of healing in the world!**

Just think of that—more people around the globe use herbal medicine on average than they use conventional medicine. Can that be a huge mistake that they use herbs? How could it possibly be?

In some areas, those who depend on botanical healing more than conventional healing lead glowing, vibrant lives. **So if there's something to herbalism, what's the big secret?** Let my book reveal that to you—and read on if you want to know.

Herbalism: A Tradition, and a History

What makes most of the world turn to herbal healing, then? What's the big secret?

Well, it's not really a secret. In essence, it is herbalism's long-standing history and tradition that win the trust of so many people. **Not to mention—it's completely natural!**

All of our ancestors turned to plants as medicine, no matter their country of origin, race, culture, creed, or religion. It's even arguable that our bodies became accustomed to and strengthened by the plants we got acquainted with over time: according to each unique culture, its medicine ways, and the evolved diets of our ancestors. This can't be said for pharmaceuticals and drugs today—filled with chemicals and substances our bodies are not used to, our ancestors never used, and which have only been around for a couple hundred years.

Anciently, expert healers in all cultures compiled, observed, and experimented with all sorts of different plants of their local region—such as shamans, medicine people, healers, priests and doctors. **It was only through thousands of years of trial, error, perfection, and teaching that herbal lore became a navigable body of medicine, which still holds value today.**

The globe has relied upon this "traditional research" for much longer than man-made medicines, even though they have been scientifically researched in their own right. **The secret**—which is not really a secret—is that traditional herbalism is arguably more popular and well-researched than mainstream healthcare in its own way.

Even better—the very basic tenets of herbalism, though thousands of years old, can be practiced by anyone to empower their health at home: to heal ailments from colds and allergies, to insomnia and headaches. There is practically no end to the herbal knowledge you can learn. You can find those basic tenets of homemade herbal medicine in the education-packed pages ahead!

My Own Herbal Journey

There are many reasons why so many are drawn to herbal medicine, and it's no coincidence, let me tell you. Even better, this book will give you all those reasons—in an easy, succinct, compact guide that can get you started on your own healing journey.

If you are just starting on the colorful road into botanical healing, I want to let you know: many years ago, I was just like you. I loved the idea of herbs, taking health into my own hands, and learning herbal traditions that were thousands of years old.

But my questions were the same. **Do herbs really work?**

Starting out, those questions led me at the time to delving into literature on my own. I decided to apprentice and study with professional master herbalists and traditional healers, in order to learn and see how herbal healing really worked.

I quickly learned that there is an enormous acumen of knowledge in herbalism, and thousands of plants out there: all with claims to fame on how they support your health and act as medicines, like they did many, many years ago before modern medicine.

The truth is: in some form, all of them really do work in some healing way. But after learning traditional methods however, I also wanted to learn the scientific take on well-established healing herbs. What did science have to say?

I quickly realized that there is a lot of controversy and misinformation over plant medicines in the mainstream health world! **Have you ever looked up herbal info online, only to not know which article is wrong, and which one is right?**

I certainly did. There was so much info in the online world, I had no idea who to believe and what information about herbalism to trust. Some claimed that herbs worked miracles, while others said that herbalism had always been nothing but quackery!

I knew that both were not fully true, especially the latter. This started me on a new journey into herbalism: finding the support of scientific studies, trials, and research on plants that *DO* in fact have proof of their effects.

Over time, I compiled my own writings and research into a guide I myself used with my loved ones—all about which herbs were the most widely respected in traditional use, science, and my own observation combined.

As I used this guide in my daily life and education, it struck me one day: **why not take what I have learned over these many years and craft it as a home health guide for all?**

It is my personal journey through herbal education, research, learning, and practice that has brought you this book today.

In the pages ahead, you will find all the basics—and ultimately the *TRUTH* of today's front-line herbal remedies. With all the research and traditional knowledge right there at your fingertips, I think you will be relieved that you don't have to do all the footwork like I did... though all of it was absolutely worth it to get this book out into the public, and finally, into your hands.

What It Means to Use Herbal Medicine

Even better than having all the information at your fingertips, is knowing exactly what to do with it. **Not only will I share with you my favorite herbal remedies and their abilities to handle all sorts of ailments, but how and when to use this knowledge as well: at home, and in your personal health regimen.**

Mastering herbal knowledge takes wisdom, caution, and informed judgement. In spite of all the knowledge in this book, there is a good time to use herbs, and there is a time to take your ailments to the professional help of a more knowledgeable, professional herbalist—or even a doctor when things get serious.

You can't handle all your health issues on your own. But you can handle your personal care, and prevent future health problems by taking the wheel with the wise use of herbs at home, where it is warranted. **This book will show you how.**

I want to thank you again for the purchase of this book I put so much work into, which I hope saves you time, money, and pain in bettering your health. If my book succeeds, I also hope to see you transform from a person with simple questions about herbs... into a person who gets as excited and devoted to learning about herbs as I am!

For the rest of you out there who already love and are passionate about herbalism: I'm sure you need no convincing or persuasion to read on, and dive into the wonderful chapters of this book—

to learn all about herbs, the remedies they enact, and especially the subjects of our very first chapter, *"Using Medicinal Plants!"*

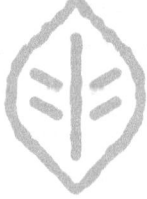

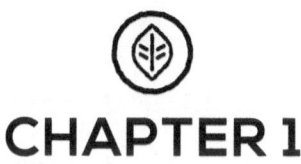

CHAPTER 1

Using Medicinal Plants

Before we get into the many helpful, healing herbs out there, a good place to start with using herbs at home is by learning their universal uses first. There are a number of methods that apply to most, if not all, plants for using them in healing at home—and this helps as a first step before approaching each individual healing plant.

Unlike modern medicine's pills, cough syrups or creams, herbs are perishable and natural. You must think of them more like healing foods that could possibly go bad, in a way.

But unlike most foods, you'll want to hold on to them longer—maximizing their storage capacity while being able to use them as quickly, easily, and conveniently as possible, when you need them.

Some herbs you'll want to purchase at your natural foods or health store, which makes storage easier (most herbal products are retailed for easier storage—such as supplements). But what about when you want to harvest herbs from the wild, in the case of "wildcrafting"—or use them from your garden or backyard?

Herbalists over millennia have perfected these techniques: whether that be the harvesting, storing, or preparation of herbs in order to make the most of their application and perishability. In the following sections, we'll find those techniques and explore the basics of how to harness nature's plant miracles.

Harvesting Herbs

What kind of plant are you wishing to harvest? Depending on the plant you're targeting, it has various parts of value that you will want to take and use at home. Each part is harvested differently, and thus must be approached differently.

Maybe it's the stems, or just the leaves of a plant, with reported healing abilities that you want to use. You could be after the buds or flowers—or perhaps you're wanting to employ a plant's root for a specific issue.

Specific parts require specific harvesting techniques. Here's the "How-to" on the general approach to each plant part—but if you are wanting to get into detail, I would recommend looking up the unique techniques specific to each medicinal herb in the upcoming sections!

Harvesting Herbs (From Top to Bottom):

• *Flowers and Buds* – In most cases, you can delicately remove flowers, buds, and petals with your fingers. Pinch the "neck" or stem of the flower, where it attaches to its branch, between the thumb and forefinger; gently remove and place in a breathable container, such as a basket, before storage. **The best time to harvest is in spring—but certain plants can vary.**

> • *If flower or bud stems are too tough, try using a clean pair of scissors or garden snippers.*

• *Berries or Fruits* – Like with flowers, fruits can be removed gently with your fingers. Using a canvas bag or metal container (like a bowl) for holding works well, and take special care if fruits "stain" easily (such as Elderberries). **Best time to harvest: late summer or fall, though it varies with plant.**

> • *Similar to flowers and buds, use clean scissors/garden snippers of removal of fruits/berries is too difficult.*

• ***Stems or Leaves ("Aerial Parts")*** – On tender-stemmed plants (such as mint or chamomile, e.g.) stems and leaves can be gently removed with a pinch and snap of the fingers. For tougher plants, use a knife, scissors, or snippers—bundle and tie together in bunches to prepare for hanging and drying, with a rubber band or hair-tie. **Best to harvest in spring or summer.**

> • *With hands or tools, you may also "clear" an entire plant in the case of annual (short-lived) plants, or those you don't want to tend to year after year. Simply cut it at the stem clear to the root, right above where it enters into the ground—but in most cases, don't expect the plant to grow back!*

• ***Twigs and Bark*** – Some herbs have healing effects found in the "inner" bark, such as on shrubs or trees. Using a specialized knife or clippers, the outermost twigs can be harvested on a living plant, which should hold the same healing properties as the bark. **Best to harvest in spring, when the sap flows.**

> • *Be careful harvesting actual bark or certain amounts of twigs from living plants, if you don't want to see them become diseased or die (especially endangered/threatened plants). It is considered more ecological to take bark from trees or shrubs that have just fallen and are expected to be deceased.*

• **Roots** – With a spade, shovel or gloves, remove the root from the ground of the desired herb you wish to use. For some plants, you can also dig down and only remove part of the root to keep the plant alive (such as with Echinacea and other endangered plants). **Best to harvest in late fall or winter.**

• **Whole Plant** – If there are many plants in the area, they are not endangered, and you plan to use all of its parts for medicine at home—use some sturdy gloves and pull it out by the root. Stubborn plant? Use the aid of a shovel or spade if a plant's roots are too strong for pulling out by hand alone!

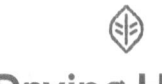

Drying Herbs

So you've harvested your plants. Now you want to hang onto your plants for long-term use and storage. What's next?

Many herbalists dry their herbs before using them at all. Especially if you are wanting to store them in "raw" form, drying is almost always necessary. Storing herbs "fresh" requires several special preparation methods—you can do that too, but we'll get to that later!

As with harvesting, each plant part you'll want to dry a little differently. Certain parts need more time than others. For each separate part, here's how.

Drying Herbs (From Top to Bottom):

• *Flowers and Buds* – Spread these evenly on an open basket or screen in one layer, with the edges of flowers barely touching (never piling up). Leave to dry for just a few days to a week in an area that is dark and dry, getting adequate air circulation—flowers mold especially easily, so this is essential!

• **Berries or Fruits** – Dry these similar to flowers or buds, laying them out in a single layer. Leave to dry somewhere with little moisture and some air circulation, such as near a fan, for a few days to a week. Some fruits can be sun-dried, others should not be. If you have a food dehydrator, it works excellently!

• **Stems or Leaves** – After bundling these after harvest, hang bundles upside down on a line (clothesline, e.g.) in a dry area for about a week. Running a fan on low can help. Wrap bundles beforehand in something like a paper bag—this prevents excess wilting, loss of healing properties due to sun damage, and the accumulation of dust or other debris in leaves while drying.

• **Barks or Twigs** – Spread evenly, only one layer thick, on a screen or basket with edges of barks twigs only barely touching. Dry in a dark place with no moisture. Barks and twigs take much longer to dry, sometimes 2 weeks to a month. Running a fan on low can help.

• **Roots** – Using a cutting board and sharp knife beforehand, cut and slice all roots open "length-wise" the entire length of the root to assist with drying. Whole roots are more susceptible to rot or slow drying, if not cut. If you so desire, roots can be "diced and cubed." Drying takes 2 weeks to a month—store in a dark, dry place until then, running a fan on low can assist with drying times.

Storing Herbs

After the drying process, dried herb parts need to be moved into some sort of storage. That way, they stay dry—or they don't get so dry and brittle that you simply can't use them anymore! In that same vein, you also want to prevent your already dry herbs from getting wet again, and possibly experiencing some mold or mildew problems.

You'll also want to store your herbs in such a way that they're easy to access, ready to use conveniently, whenever you want.

The following are tried-and-true herbal storing methods. Whether you have dried leaves, stems, roots or twigs, most herbs can simply be broken up by hand and stored in the following containers.

Want great-looking tea blends, herb mixes or powders? Try using a mortar and pestle to grind up your herbs before placing them into your desired container. It's a lot of work, but makes your dried stores look great!

Also try sifting leaves and stems through a screen or strainer for a finer-looking tea, or even a powder you can add or mix into foods and soups.

- *Glass Jars* – This is the most popular among herbalists. Dried plant parts of most kinds do very well in glass containers (save for flowers and berries), with a lid to screw on and protect from moisture or dust.

  - *Opt for dark colored glass, like amber, green or blue— these also help protect your dried herbs from light damage, which sap away the healing compounds!*

• **_Stainless Steel Metal Containers_** – These work exceptionally well too, and automatically protect plants from sun damage. Berries and some flowers do a little better stored in metal containers than in glass—where they are prone to mold.

• **_Paper Bags_** – Herb parts that are the most susceptible to mold or mildew fare the best in paper bags, as paper helps naturally wick away damaging moisture. Brown paper bags further assist in protecting from damaging light. Certain herb leaves, flowers, and berries store much better in here than anywhere else.

• **_Plastic Baggies_** – The use of plastic can, of course, be controversial. If it's the only thing you have access to, it works pretty well. If you are concerned about harmful plastic substances leeching into your herbs—such as BPA's and xenoestrogens—then opt for something different, or try as often as possible to store plastic bags of herbs away from sunlight.

Kept and stored well, you can hang on to your dried herbs and tea blends for 1-2 years. If herbs are looking brown and dull, with no fresh scent, it's time to chuck them out and harvest more.

Herbal Preparations

Harvesting, drying, and storing your herbs is really only the first step on a multi-faceted path of using herbs. Of course, the above methods are only the practical part—now it's time to get into using them for yourself, to boost your health!

Teas, Infusions, Tisanes and Compresses

Ever made your very own herbal tea before? How about to promote a little herbal healing in your life? Chances are you already have. Maybe without even really knowing it!

Once you have built up your very own stores of dried herbs, you'll have a wide assortment of loose-leaf teas to choose from. It helps to buy your own tools for making loose leaf tea at home with your own dried herbs, with the help of **tea balls, tea strainers or even "infusers."**

"Wait—what are 'tisanes' and 'compresses?'" Yes, we're getting into some more complex herbalist terminology here. But realize that a "tisane" and a "compress," even an "infusion," are all basically just teas. Simply think of them as teas you use in different ways!

- *Tea* – Take 1 tsp to 1 tbsp. of your desired dried herb, and steep in boiled water for 5 minutes. Sip or make multiple cups for mild ailments and symptoms.

- *Infusion* – Take 1 to 5 tbsps. of your desired dried herb, and steep in boiled water for 15-20 minutes. If you so like, you can actually boil the herb for 15-20 minutes in the water itself—before straining off and drinking. Infusions are great for slightly more acute ailments and symptoms.

- *Tisane* – This can also be called a "wash." Using the exact same methods for making an infusion, use the infusion itself as a topical wash for hair, eyes, and skin. Great for cosmetic uses, or to rinse out the eyes.

- *Compress* – Another topical use of teas and infusions, compresses involve taking a clean cloth, soaking it in the infusion, and applying it to maladies like burns, boils, cuts, bruises, or skin afflictions (such as eczema).

For using teas and infusions for various ailments, typically drink 2-3 cups/per day from about 1 tsp to 1 Tbsp. of the dried plant with most plants—unless otherwise noted with certain plants in the chapters ahead, for safety's sake.

Oils and Salves

This is where herbal preparations become more elaborate and complicated. But these are also excellent beginning preparations to learn, if you are just starting out—and very fun to use!

Oils – Take your chosen dried herb, and place it in a jar. Cover the dried herb with a food-safe oil of your choice: safflower, sunflower, and avocado are popular choices (organic and cold pressed or expeller pressed are considered best for the body!)

• **Place on a windowsill with some exposure to sunlight, and let herbal properties infuse into the oil for about a week.** Once done, strain herb matter from oil completely, and store in a bottled/lidded glass jar out of the sunshine.

• **Or:** place oil and herb matter in a small saucepan, and heat up on very low heat until oil changes color (as it absorbs herbs qualities). **Only opt for an oil with a high smoke point if using this method.** Once infused, let cool, then strain herb matter into bottled/lidded glass jar for storage.

• **You can also use fresh herbs to infuse into your oil, not just dried.** However, if using fresh herbs, avoid consuming/using these oils internally!

• **With dried herb-infused oils**, you can use sprinkled on food, or add it to salad dressings for healing effects. **For any infused oil**, you can take a teaspoon or two and rub onto (closed) skin for pains, aches, moisturizing, or other benefits!

How long can I store or keep my oil? Kept in a dark, cool place away from sunlight—and made correctly—oils can be fresh at least 1 year. Throw them out if they go rancid—if they suddenly take on a nutty or plastic smell, they've gone bad and shouldn't be used.

Salves – The next step up from oils, salves are a lot easier to make than they might sound. All it involves is heating up an herbal oil, adding beeswax or a vegetable-based wax (such as candelilla or carnuba, for example), and letting that harden into a "balm" you pour out into separate jars.

   • **Simply make your desired oil** – when complete, heat oil up in a small saucepan (or the top of a double-burner, if you have one) on low, and only use herbal oils that have a high smoke point.

   • **Add anywhere from 1 tsp to 1 tbsp. of all-natural, clean wax to the oil (I prefer to use a cruelty free vegetable-based wax).** Watch wax melt, stir if you like. Take note that for salves made with candelilla oil, you won't need to add nearly as much wax.

      • *"Balmy" or "Oily" Salve? Dip in a knife, stick, or small spoon into the heated oil and place in the freezer for a minute. Take it out, and you can gauge the consistency of what the salve will be like when it's cooled.*

         - *Too Oily?* Just add more wax.

         - *Too Balmy?* Is your salve more like a candle-stick? You might then have to add more oil—or next time, add less wax and work up to the consistency you want.

- **Set up several clean, open containers on the side that will hold your salves.** *Glass or stainless steel work best—and make sure each container has a lid!*

- **Pour salve (with wax all melted and stirred in) into each jar.** *Let each jar sit and cool in a place where they cannot be bumped, or stuff can fall into and ruin the salve.*

- **Once oil and wax is solidified, you have jars of salve!** *Apply it to your skin to moisturize, or to healing wounds or burns once they have closed. Not happy with the consistency? Try adding a different amount of wax next time.*

As with oils, well-made salves remain unperishable for at least a year.

Tinctures and Vinegars

In this realm, you're moving up to the level of more professional, practical herbalists! For both dried and fresh herbs alike, tinctures and vinegars can be excellent for long-term storage—lasting much longer than dried herbs, infusions, salves or oils.

Each of these preparations either incorporates alcohol (tinctures) or vinegar, which prolong preservation... a very old trick learned and passed down among herbalists. This helps the herbs you harvested last longer, and in some ways, makes their use a bit more fast and convenient.

Vinegars – Similar to making an infused oil, fill a clean jar with your choice dry or fresh herb. Cover your herb completely with vinegar—white or apple cider vinegars both work well, then lid the jar.

• **Store in a dark, cool place for about a week.** The refrigerator works quite well. Feel free to shake sporadically, which helps break up the herb matter and impart its qualities into the vinegar better.

• **If you are using a metal lid,** it is wise to add a "liner" of wax paper before screwing it on when infusing vinegars. This is because: vinegar slowly eats away at metal over time!

• **Once "steeped," strain out herbal matter and store in separate glass container in your fridge.** Again—if you're capping this container with something metal, make sure to line it so the vinegar doesn't eat the metal away! Use this vinegar in topical applications, like a tincture, or even as a salad dressing.

Tinctures – Like with infusing vinegars, instead one pours alcohol over their selected herbs. This helps you save your herbs for an extended period of time—some say the herbs stay good up to 10 years. Sometimes even forever!

• **It is best to select a high-proof alcohol for your tincture,** to absorb as many plant constituents as possible. Brandy or Vodka is popular, although "Everclear" is considered the very best. Higher-proof, the better!

• **Store in a dark, cool place for at least 2 weeks to 2 months.** Shake once in a while, like with herbal vinegars.

• **Once time is up, strain out your tincture.** Bottle it in smaller containers—or you can even get "dropper" bottles so you can administer your tincture in small doses or drops.

• **Using Your Tincture** – For most of the herbs discussed in this book, doses for any illness is **2-3 droppers per day**, until issues recede—or follow the specific guidance given for each herb in the next few chapters.

Purchasing Your Herbs

Admittedly, purchasing herbs becomes necessary in some cases. The adventurous herbalist or first-timer may get more delight out of drying herbs and making their own preparations at home—but it is simply better and more called for sometimes to get to your natural food store, grocer, herbalist or apothecary to see what's out there.

Why, exactly? There are a number of reasons why you should stick to buying certain herbs or herbal preparations:

• **It is best to take them in supplement or essential oil form.** Some teas or tinctures of specific herbs are incredibly bitter, so you have to figure out a pleasant way to get them in you—that's what **supplements** are for.

> • *In some instances too,* **capsuled herbs**—*usually containing a small bit of the freeze-dried leaves, herbs, roots, or flowers—works better than other preparations (as in the case of Nettle supplements for allergies, or Goldenseal for digestive issues).*

> • *Some herbs come commonly, or* **only** *in* **essential oil** *form (Eucalyptus and Tea Tree are good examples). If you want to work with these herbs, you will have to use them as essential oils—but even further, learn the proper ways of using essential oils for healing.*

• **The herbs are rare, endangered, or threatened, and you should not harvest them—but instead seek them out from an ethical, sustainable grower or harvester.**

> • *Some good examples include* **Echinacea, Goldenseal,** *and* **Black Cohosh**. *It's best you get to the grocer and buy dried or powdered herb, supplements, or tinctures*

from reputable buyers who can trustingly say they are not damaging the plant's population permanently.

Buying Essential Oils

Perhaps you are dealing with more of a topical skin issue, such as Athlete's Foot or a minor wound. Maybe you would like to soothe a headache, or simply have a calming aroma in your home.

In that case, purchasing essential oils could be a perfect fit. **Some words of caution though:**

• **Ensure to only use high-quality essential oils, *NOT* toxic 'fragrance' oils.** These cheap imitations are worse than ineffective. They actually fill your body and brain with neurotoxins, making you feel headachy, stressed and anxious.

• **Always look for the words '100% pure essential oil' on the label.** Choose glass bottles that are dark blue, green or brown to make sure they will last.

• **As a general rule for skin application, every 1 drop of essential oil should be diluted with at least 5ml of carrier oil or other fluid** (with the exception of a few essential oils that can be used 'neat' or direct onto the skin)

   • *Some common carrier oil types that are affordable and easy to find include:* **sweet almond oil, olive oil, sunflower oil, coconut oil, castor oil, jojoba oil and avocado oil.**

• **Do not ingest essential oils and keep out of reach of children and pets.**

• **Ensure essential oils do not come into contact with your eyes and open wounds, and use with caution if**

you are pregnant, planning to become pregnant, or have any pre-existing medical conditions.

• If you have any sensitivities or concerns about using essential oils, ensure you try a patch test first.

Buying Herbal Supplements

There are many companies, brands, and stores out there that sell herbal supplements for health, wellness, and acute issues. My best advice to anyone shopping the supplement-path: **always purchase supplements from companies with an expansive, good reputation, ethical harvesting and growing practices, and organically-grown or foraged plants.**

What's the true advantage of getting herbs into your life in supplement form? Well, let's take a look at some of the pros and cons.

Pros:

• **You don't have to taste them.** It's true: some very powerful herbs you might really want in your life, such as **Goldenseal** and **Reishi**, taste awful to most. Fortunately, supplements give you the chance to not always pass them up.

• **You don't have to look for or harvest them.** Reputable supplement companies do the job for you, especially with difficult-to-find, even rare and endangered plants. Unless you love the outdoors, this could skip you a trip traipsing through the woods.

  • *Some herbs you might not be able to find in your country or area at all.* ***Turmeric, Ginger,*** *and* ***Ashwagandha*** *are enviable herbs, but they grow only in Asia profusely.*

What if you don't live in Asia? Supplement companies help some of these plants become readily available to you.

• **Supplements retain the freshness and healing qualities of certain plants better than any other preparation.** Stinging Nettle is a good example, along with Cayenne, Echinacea, or Evening Primrose (in supplement "oil" form). The preparations you make at home just couldn't do nearly as much, if you notice—so opt for the supplement route.

Cons:

• **Some supplement companies are untrustworthy.** Make sure you stick to widely reputable, trusted supplement companies—recent studies into supplements found that many were filled with "adulterants," or herbs and matter that definitely did not match the advertiser's label.

  • ***Want to make sure your herbs work?*** *Make your own stuff, pure and simple.*

• **You don't form a relationship with nature, the plant, or have a connection with your medicine.** This might not be a concern to you at all—and you simply want a more natural, convenient form of healing. But if you really want to feel more connected to your food, nutrition and healing—much like you might want to get more acquainted with your food through gardening, etc.—supplements will not provide that so much.

For using supplements at home, always follow the directions on the product label.

Creams and Ointments

Similar in scope to supplements and essential oils, some powerful medicinal herbs work best only in commercially made, fairly available creams, gels or ointments.

You could try to make these same creams and ointments in salve or oil form, but they may just not be as effective. **Cayenne** creams, more specifically called *capsaicin* creams, are one good example—they are formulated and crafted specifically so they can be used in a safe, easy, and highly beneficial way.

As we explore specific healing herbs more deeply, some will be noted that they only come in commercial ointments or creams. If you are the more advanced herbalist—maybe you could foray into the world of home-made ointment or cream making. But for the beginner, see if a store-bought cream or ointment satisfies you enough—there's always time for inspiration later!

For using commercial creams and ointments at home, always follow the directions and product label.

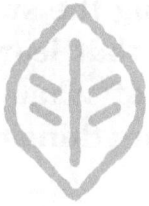

CHAPTER 2

The Top 5 Essential Herbs and their Uses

A newcomer to the world of herbal healing might be overwhelmed by the sheer volume of herbs out there. Over the ages, hundreds if not thousands of plants have been used for all sorts of ailments in traditional medicine and other practices: headaches, colds, skin afflictions, belly aches, you name it.

Today, a way of universally navigating that information is lost. Modern medicine and mainstream research are only themselves just beginning to catch up on understanding herbalism, and to navigate this sea of useful botanical information in a way that can be grasped easily by all.

Even then, there is still controversy about the use of herbs and what they do exactly, which study today strives to clarify. What ancient cultures' herbal practitioners once documented and passed on is only known and kept by a few, and in a fragmented way that lacks the scientific approach.

Even after just scratching the surface of herbalism as a beginner, you realize that learning the art involves knowing all the facets of what each plant does—but where to begin without anything to guide you?

I'll tell you, even an herb nut like me had to start somewhere! **But I'll share with you my little trick I used to gain footing in the herbal world—I learned the uses, effects, and powers of 5 herbs that were the most studied and widely supported for common ailments.**

Even more, I selected 5 that would cover the widest range of ailments possible, so I only had to start with 5 for practically all my at-home uses. I then perfected my knowledge and uses with each of them, and from there, used the first 5 to branch out to the rest of the herbal world!

With this I open up our next chapter: *The Top 5 Essential Herbs and their Uses*. These are the first 5 herbs I studied when I started out. I got acquainted with each intimately, learned all the many studies supporting them, as well as gleaned all the traditional information on their classical healing effects.

Now you too can use these 5 as a starting point. If you're bold enough and love herbs, you can then delve into our next section, which will explore the uses of so many more.

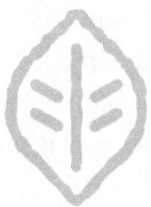

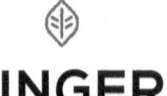

GINGER

(Zingiber officinalis)

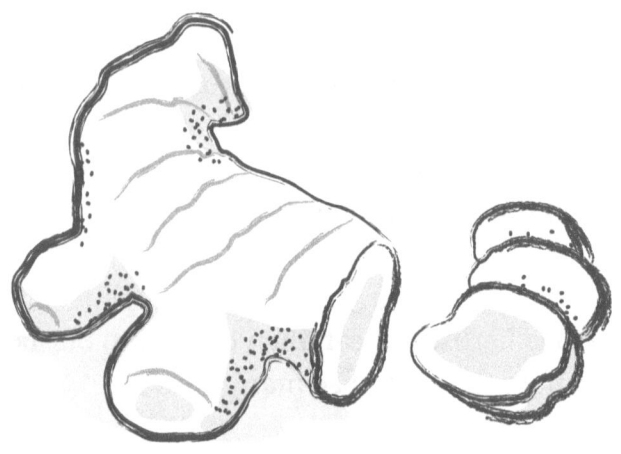

Your cold-fighter, stomach soother, and anti-inflammatory

Hailing from Asia, Ginger not only found it's way into delicious ethnic cuisine—it was also used for its powerful healing effects. Traditional herbalists and scientists alike have noticed its usefulness to fight colds, aid digestion, and allay the pains of inflammation. Consider Ginger a must-have to begin your at-home healing regimen. Even if it's not in use for its effects—have it on hand to add a taste of the East to your meals! ***Make sure to exercise caution and avoid using large amounts of Ginger daily with pregnant women, small children, and some with heartburn disorders.***

Supports Colds and Flu – Chinese studies in-vitro showed compounds in Ginger being able to **kill viruses**. Taking Ginger could help you or a loved one get through a cold all the quicker. Indian studies revealed that Ginger can **help ramp up the immune system** in response to colds and flus.

Ginger is a powerful anti-inflammatory. Consuming the root can help soothe inflammation of the sinuses, throat, lungs, and respiratory passageways in colds.

Digestive Aid – Ginger might be most famous for helping with **nausea**. Even the National Cancer Institute observed Ginger in chemo-therapy patients reducing nausea symptoms by another 40% with conventional medications!

As a powerful **anti-inflammatory**, Ginger can be used to allay pain and inflammation in the digestive tract due to heartburn or ulcers. Ginger is also an **anti-spasmodic**. It is approved in some European countries for stomach cramps, and is even powerful enough for female complaints.

Anti-Inflammatory – This Asian root's effects against inflammation are so strong, some arthritis and rheuatism journal studies have tested its influence on joint pain for osteo-arthritis. Apparently, some of its effects can be compared to those of NSAID's like Ibuprofen and Aspirin!

Home Remedy Use: If experiencing any of the above ailments, try a Ginger tea or infusion. 1 Tbsp of Ginger powder or chopped root will do, a couple of times a day.

You can also store Ginger long-term for use in a tincture or vinegar. Try applying a compress for joint pain and issues, or add Ginger to an oil or salve, either as culinary powder or in essential oil form. You can also experience Ginger's healing effects by adding it to your food, purchasing it in supplement form, or finding it in one of its favorite store-bought forms: ginger ale!

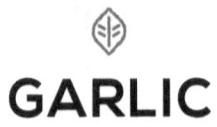

GARLIC

(Allium sativa)

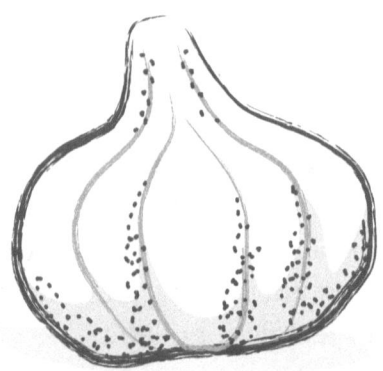

Immune-booster, natural antibiotic, and blood pressure ally

It's no coincidence that some of the most popular culinary spices are some of nature's healing miracles at the same time. Garlic is esteemed as a medicinal plant all over the world, in myriads of cultures, and is the very proof and poster-child of this phenomena. While it originates from western Russia near the Caucasus Mountains, its powers were so obvious and noticeable that Garlic found its way into the cuisine and herbalism traditions of ancient China, Rome, Greece, Egypt, the Middle East, and Europe. **Please be wary of its use if you have a blood clotting disorder, or take anticoagulants.**

Stimulates the Immune System — Garlic's influence on the immune system is astounding. Not only is Garlic's active ingredient, allicin, a **confirmed anti-oxidant** of enviable intensity—but studies on AIDS patients have shown incredible immune enhancement after daily doses of garlic cloves!

• Such a powerful stroke on the immune system has also made Garlic a front-line, long-time remedy against colds, flus, respiratory viruses and other infections.

Natural Antibiotic – Garlic's active ingredient allicin has amazing purported antimicrobial capabilities. Not only can it kill bacteria, it has been observed as an **anti-fungal, anti-viral, and anti-protozoan**.

• Tests and tradition together have seen Garlic actively combat infections such as amoebic dysentery, salmonella, E. Coli infection, tuberculosis, athlete's food, women's yeast infections, and even the viral flu.

• Garlic's active compount allicin is only formed when Garlic is crushed or chopped, and then quickly oxidizes. As such, its immune-boosting and antibiotic effects together can only be attained by eating fresh, chopped Garlic quickly.

Blood Pressure and Cholesterol – Allicin and another garlic compound, ajoene, have been rightfully suspected as making Garlic a heart-healthy food and healing herb. In daily amounts, garlic consumption helps lower blood pressure and reduce cholesterol, as well as preventing build up of plaque and blood clots in blood vessels.

Home Remedy Use: Crush cloves for use as a topical antibiotic or anti-fungal on the skin. Crush, chop, or even chew up to even 10 garlic cloves a day to experience powerful anti-oxidant, immune-boosting and blood-pressure/cholesterol lowering effects. **Beware: fresh garlic creates a sting, and might even cause a rash/dermatitis in those sensitive.**

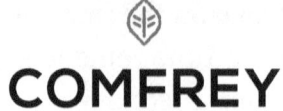

COMFREY

(Symphytum officinale)

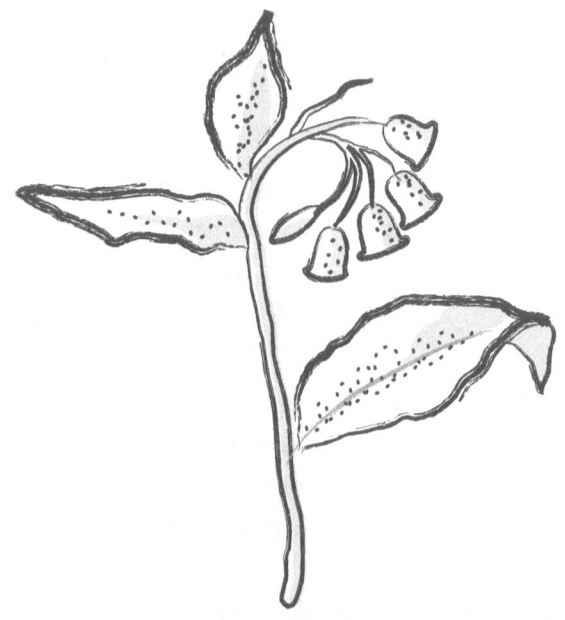

Topical magic for bone and muscle aches, sprains, bruises or breaks

In ancient Europe, Comfrey also touted names like "knitbone" and "bruisewort" for its amazing capability of helping the body bounce back from tissue damage. Applications of the fresh leaf or root, plant juices, salves, or ointments were powerful at mending minor bruises, all the way to speeding healing of broken bones. For a wide variety of herbalists today, Comfrey is an absolute must-have as a healer of the musculo-skeletal system. **Internal use is not recommended due to liver-damaging pyrrolizidine alkaloids. Topical use is determined to be absolutely safe.**

Bone, Joint, and Muscle Pain – Traditional herbalists used topical applications on unbroken skin to alleviate pains and aches of the muscles and skeletal system. Comfrey contains rosmarinic acid, a plant component observed to ease inflammation and pain alike.

• Comfrey's effects in this realm are the most studied of all—a German collection of studies observes the plant's ability to take the edge off of pain, particularly in those with back pain, arthritis, or discomfort from fractures, sprains, breaks.

Speeds the Healing of Tissues – Another constituent of Comfrey, called allantoin, is responsible for shortening healing time in bodily tissues. Using it on unbroken skin over pulled muscles, bruises, fractures or breaks has been observed cutting down on recuperation.

• Comfrey has also been determined as safe for applying to open, minor wounds. A tea or tincture could be excellent for this. Comfrey is also a common ingredient in various over-the-counter wound care creams.

Home Remedy Use: One can grind or chop up the leaves of Comfrey and apply it as a poultice to minor cuts or wounds. The same can be done by applying to the skin near fractures, bone breaks, or muscle pain. Comfrey root is also purported to have many healing compounds like rosmarinic acid and allantoin.

You can also use Comfrey in a tea or infusion as a compress for the same purpose. Comfrey oils and salves make wonderful topical applications where there is no broken skin involved.

The crafting of a Comfrey tincture or vinegar might help you store it for longer and to apply as a "liniment" in the same way, but **any preparation of Comfrey should not be taken internally for long periods of time due to risk of liver damage.**

LEMON BALM

(Melissa officinalis)

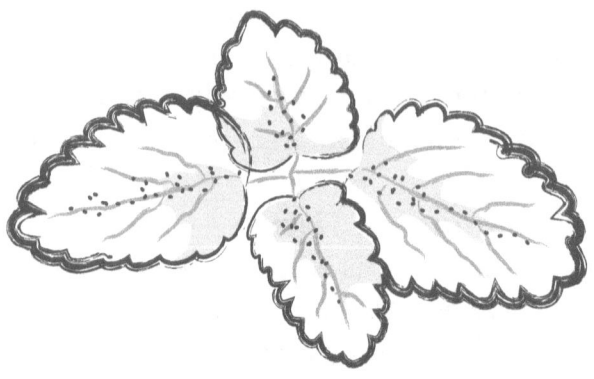

A belly-soother, tension tamer, and female ally

Think of a plant like spearmint: lush, plentiful, and cooling. Then combine it with a brush of lemony taste. You have Lemon Balm: an excellent remedy for nerves, stress, anxiety, headaches, and disturbances that can arise in female health. Its fragrance is heavenly—a crush of the leaves can untangle unrest in just moments. In Europe, this aroma was imparted and extracted to waters, tinctures, and teas to pull away the distractions of frayed nerves in old times. Its powers were also able to uplift digestive troubles, promote sleep, and support female menstrual cycles. **Avoid excess use if you have hypothryoid issues, or are pregnant.**

Fights Nervousness – Studies have approved the use of Lemon Balm in Europe for low-grade nervous issues. Lemon Balm is very helpful with **insomnia**, especially if combined with another sleep-promoter, **Valerian**. Some research proved it was just as effective as some pharmaceuticals for sleep problems.

It's been found that topical Lemon Balm essential oil helps calm moods in the elderly with dementia; in Alzheimer's patients, the plant eased agitation and improve focus, making it a powerful nervine ally.

• A study of nearly 100 breast-fed babies found that Lemon Balm consumed by the mother helped alleviate colic and crying time compared to a placebo.

• Even a nice, piping hot tea has been traditionally effective for heightened anxiety and nervousness. Even better, Lemon Balm can help settle digestive upset ("butterflies in the stomach") that arises from the jitters.

Woman's Medicine – European researchers noticed an effect of Lemon Balm on uterine muscle. It is thus thought that it could help allay menstrual cramps, as well as regulate menstrual cycles in a healthier way if taken during certain times of the month.

Hyperthyroidism – Lemon Balm has been observed lowering thyroid function. It is possible that it could help those with hyperthyroid issues alleviate their symptoms.

Viral Infections – European research has also elucidated Lemon Balm as an antiviral, making it a potnetial ally for fighting colds, flus, and even herpes or supporting HIV.

Home Remedy Use: Teas and infusions of Lemon Balm, taken daily, do exceptionally well—use 1 Tbsp dried herb per cup of water for colds, frayed nerves, women's complaints, cramps or digestive issues. Essential oils, or just a dab of tea or Lemon Balm tincture, can be added to herpes cold sores to clear them up—or to skin in other areas simply to create calm.

ASHWAGANDHA

(Withania somnifera)

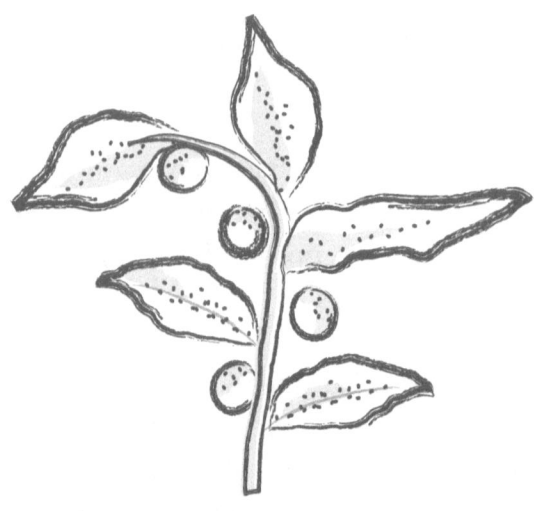

A nutritive tonic for sexual health, energy, and well-being

Ashwagandha has been a pride of India traditional herbalism and Ayurveda for centuries. Not many may know that this plant with a pungent odor—and roots rich in iron, magnesium, and other minerals—is actually very closely related to our culinary foods of the Nightshade family. These include Tomatoes, Peppers, Potatoes, and Eggplants. With such a reputation, some have called the plant "Indian Ginseng" because of its almost "cure-all" capabilities. However, Ashwagandha is more ecologically sustainable to grow, and remains a non-threatened plant, while Ginseng is neither of those things. This cornerstone of Indian herbalism also has more soothing, affirming qualities as opposed to Ginseng's more stimulant nature. **Make sure to not use this herb if pregnant, have Nightshade allergies, or if you are taking thyroid medication.**

Nutritive Tonic and Adaptogen – Research in Asian countries promotes Ashwagandha as an "adaptogen." Meaning that it contains compounds, antioxidants, vitamins and minerals that boost the immune system, protect the body from nervous or oxidative damage, withstand stress. and increase the body's ability to create energy and vitality. Over time, Ashwagandha visibly slows "cortisol" levels that lead to stress or depression by helping modulate adrenal output. Thus, this herbal medicine can be a great tonic for stress and depression over time.

• Ashwagandha extracts have been shown to influence chronic inflammation beneficially, and heal pain from osteo- and rheumatoid arthritis.

• Due to its high iron levels especially, Ashwagandha can be very nourishing, espeically for those with anxiety, depleted digestive systems, or anemia.

Sexual Health – Not only has this powerful Asian plant evidenced boosts in energy and well-being, sexual health appears to benefit particularly from Ashwagandha. A trial of about 100 adults given the herb or the placebo showed improvement not only in energy levels, but libido and sexual energy as well!

Thyroid Health – Evidence highly suggests that Ashwagandha stimulates thyroid activity. It could thus be beneficial for those with hypothryoid problems—but should be contraindicated in those with hyperthyroidism or who take thyroid-increasing medication.

Home Remedy Use: Drink an Ashwagandha infusion or tea up to 3 times per day, using about 1 tsp of the root. Tinctures and supplements are also popularly used with this Asian herb for more convenience in daily regimens.

CHAPTER 3

25 Other Must-Have Herbal Allies

In my practice and experience, my *Top 5 Herbs* selections tend to cover all my home-healing bases time and time again. Whether it relates to aches, cramps, nerves, or bruises—almost anything, really—I can usually turn to one of my fabulous five without a second thought. All their effects are well-studied, trusted, even versatile and far-reaching, covering a wide variety of ailments, troubles and injuries. With some luck and practice, I'm sure they'll become your trusted allies, too!

But once in a while, you need another support herb (or two!) to cover your tail. Maybe one of these Top 5 just isn't doing the trick, and needs a helping herb to go the extra mile. That, or you've run out your favorite go-to herb in your herbal cabinet, cupboard, or growing at-home apothecary.

What do you do? The answer—turn to one of the 25 following herbs I value as first-rate healers, with just as much study and traditional reputation as my top 5 to support their at-home use! You might not always need them—but knowing they're there, and what they do, will be comfort enough.

ALFALFA
(Medicago sativa)

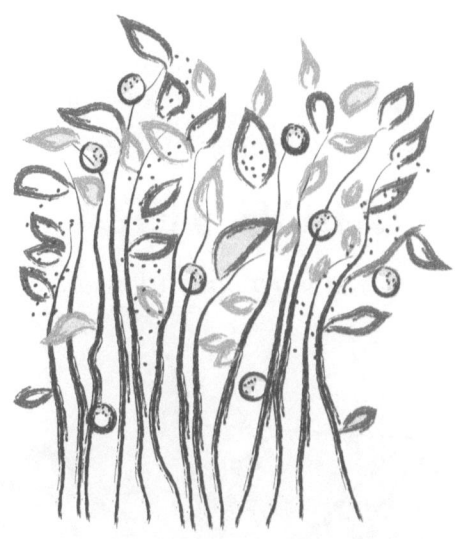

A digestive cleanser, tonic, and nutritious food and medicine

Enjoy Alfalfa sprouts? Both studies and traditional medicine hold that Alfalfa can have healing effects that combat cancer and digestive ailments. **Use Alfalfa by eating it as sprouts or leaves raw in meals, or use fresh leaves in a thick infusion every day. Alfalfa is typically available as an over-the-counter supplement as well.**

• Alfalfa is a very cleansing **digestive detoxifier** to the gut. Research observed Alfalfa binding to carcinogens in the colon. European studies suggest regular consumption of Alfalfa helps **lower cholesterol.**

• Alfalfa leaves are a significant source of **Vitamin K, Potassium, Iron, Zinc** and **Protein**, as well as Vitamins A,

B1, B6, C, and E.

Never consume Alfalfa seeds especially in high amounts daily, as they will lead to developing a blood clotting disorder.

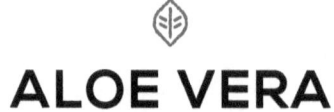

ALOE VERA

(Aloe Vera barbadensis)

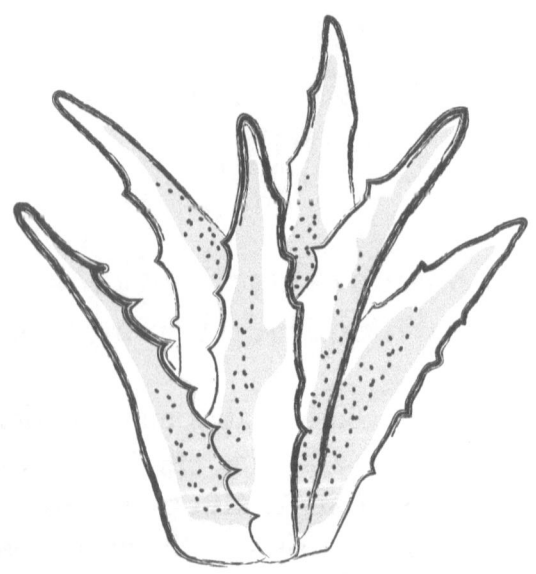

Healing for skin, wounds, burns, and Diabetics alike

You probably recognize the word "Aloe" from skin products like lotion and moisturizer. Interestingly, Aloe Vera doesn't only aid skin beauty—it heals burns, manages blood sugar, and can have some beneficial digestive effects. **Apply Aloe gel or product to skin for wounds, dryness or burns—or incorporate**

it into a salve or oil. Aloe juice can be drunk freely for helping stabilize blood sugar.

• Aloe Vera is famous for healing and relieving dry, inflamed, or itchy skin, as in cases of **psoriasis or eczema**. It excels regeneration of cells in wounds and burnt skin, including sunburns.

• Modern data suggests that Aloe can internally help lower blood sugar in type 2 Diabetics, and both internally and externally help speed diabetic wound healing.

Be cautious if taking internal Aloe products. Make sure you are only using juice or gel that is free of the latex and anthraquinones, which can cause severe digestive imbalance and diarrhea from its laxative effects.

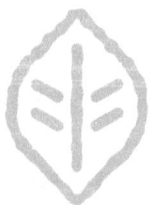

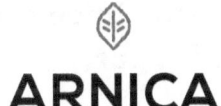

ARNICA

(Arnica montana)

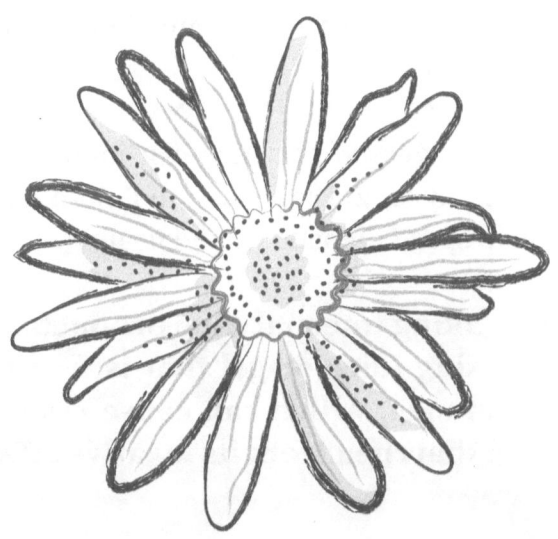

A sunny healer for bruises, muscle aches, sprains and arthritis

A dainty, humble daisy-like flower that loves mountain terrain and the Northern hemisphere, Arnica is an incredibly popular topical healer in Europe, with popularity catching up in America. **Use the dried flower heads in oils, salves, or tinctures for applying to skin where muscles, bones, or joints are sore. Or, visit your local natural food or medicine section—Arnica creams and ointments tend to be popular and plenty!**

• Applying Arnica **relieves pain and swelling** greatly in bruises, contusions, or muscular injuries where the skin is *not* open. This is due to observed **sesquiterpene lactones** thought to activate and intensely fight inflammation.

• Teas, tisanes, or liniments (in tincture or vinegar form) can

be applied to areas in need of musculoskeletal pain relief. The flower heads can also be heated and bruised as a poultice.

Never take Arnica internally or put the product on open skin, such as wounds or burns. It can cause heart and respiratory problems if absorbed into bloodstream.

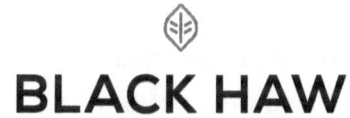

BLACK HAW

(Viburnum prunifolium)

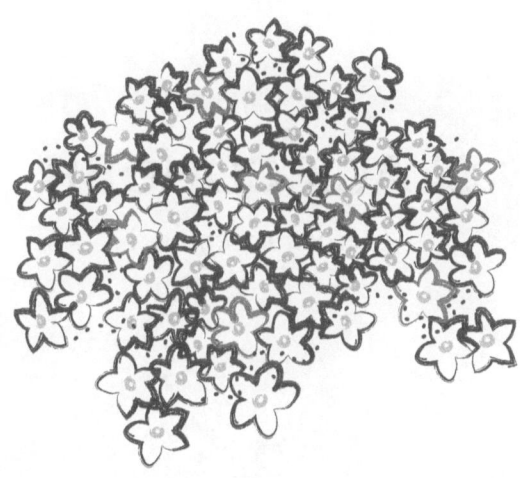

Your remedy for cramps - of all kinds

This beautiful bush—with bright red berries and cream-colored flowers—is a cornerstone favorite in United States Southern herbalism. It was once used for all sorts of women's health issues by Native Americans, even for childbirth, miscarriage, and labor. Now, it has settled into the comfortable role of allaying uterine cramps that accompany menstruation—but anyone, man or woman, can enjoy its ability to take away intestinal or stomach cramps as well. **Try a tea of dried root or stem, simmered** for about 10 minutes, or you can make or buy your own tincture. Black Haw supplements are also widely available.

• A compound in the roots and stems called scopoletin works to soothe spasms in smooth muscles, whether found in the digestive tract or uterus. It also works on smooth muscle in the trachea, making Black Haw beneficial for **asthma symptoms and attacks**.

Black Haw should not be used in women who are pregnant, nor in children under 16 or those with Aspirin allergies.

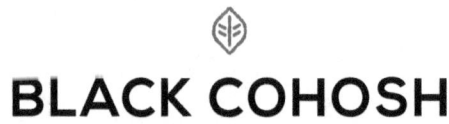

BLACK COHOSH

(Actaea racemosa)

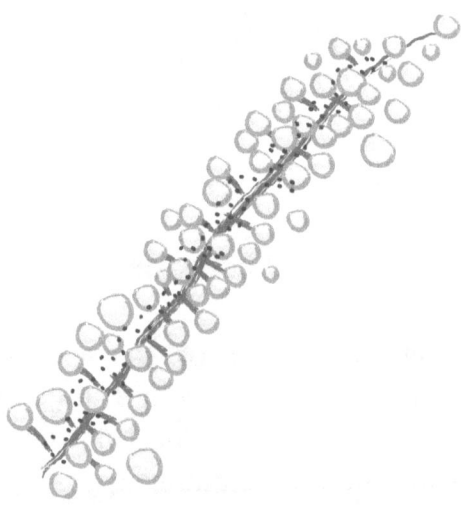

Nature's healing hormonal resource
for women

A native to North America, this stunning plant (once used for snakebites in Native herbalism) has become an important herbal medicine for women today. It contains compounds called "phytoestrogens," which mimic estrogen and fit perfectly in female hormone receptors. **Supplements or tincture of Black Cohosh root are the most popular, taken every day for certain female complaints. If you have access to ecologically harvested root yourself, consider making your own homemade tincture, or a hot tea daily (use ½ to 1 Tbsp. per cup).**

• Some herbalists say Black Cohosh is good for women with menstrual problems. It is more precisely relieving for women with low estrogen levels: especially women in **menopause**. It can provide a natural hormonal replacement therapy, but check with your physician.

• Some menstrual issues are in fact due to low estrogen. If you have PCOS (Polycystic Ovarian Syndrome), adult acne issues and/or irregular menses, consider getting your hormone levels checked and trying Black Cohosh.

Avoid Black Cohosh if you are pregnant, and make sure you are taking Black Cohosh, not *Blue* Cohosh, which can be dangerous. Avoid taking it if you have a liver disease.

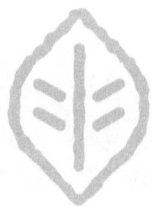

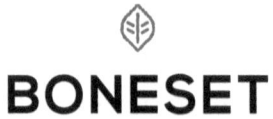

BONESET

(Eupatorium perfoliaturn)

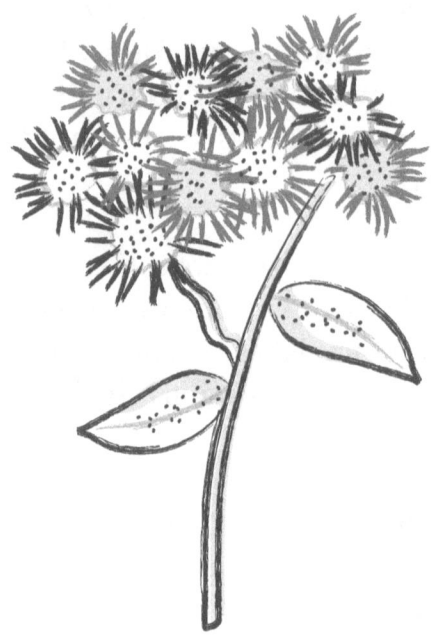

A Colds and Flu Remedy - not to be overlooked

It might be hard not to think this plant has something to do with bones. But actually, its ancient, old-time use was for alleviating colds, flus, and fevers so intense that they literally made your bones hurt! **Use the *dried* leaves of this towering plant in a hot tea or tincture, and take daily for the duration of minor viral illnesses.**

• Before modern medicine, Boneset was used to fight Dengue fever and cases of Malaria that wouldn't respond to quinine bark—making it highly reputable to colds with fevers.

• Studies claim that Boneset's effects on colds and flu are due to increased stimulation of white blood cells, which help fight off foreign infection.

Do not use the plant fresh, in large amounts, or every day for the long-term. It causes diarrhea, nausea, vomiting, and liver damage. It contains pyrrolizidine alkaloids, much like Comfrey, when used fresh or often.

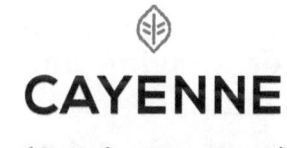

CAYENNE

(Capsicum anuum)

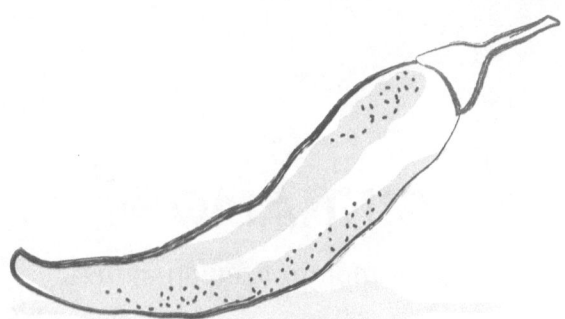

A spicy food, digestive aid, and topical nerve pain reliever

Some believe Cayenne and other hot peppers damage the stomach (and your skin) in high amounts due to spicy chemicals. That is a myth—this Southwestern pepper's active ingredient, *capsaicin*, is actually helpful for digestion and relieves pain for some issues. **Add Cayenne powder or chopped pepper to your food to feel its effects—or you can easily obtain supplements. Over-the-counter pain relief creams with capsaicin are also available for topical pain issues.**

• Capsaicin creams, added topically to **unbroken** skin, have showed great improvement for joint, muscle, and peripheral nerve pains. Its benefits could aid those with osteoarthritis, fibromyalgia, sciatica, and even diabetic neuropathy.

• Cayenne pepper has been shown to stimulate saliva flow and gastric juices, helping the body break down food more efficiently.

Discontinue use of Cayenne/capsaicin products if redness, burning, or stinging on the skin occurs no matter what after multiple uses. Some irritation is normal at first, however. Do not apply to open, broken skin.

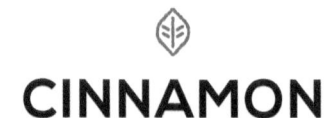

CINNAMON

(Cinnamomum zeylonicum)

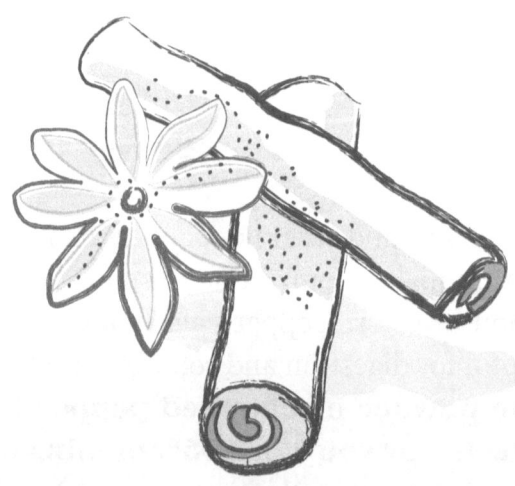

Sweet spice for sweet problems -
Diabetes and cholesterol

Ironically, this spice commonly found with sweet foods happens to be excellent at blood sugar control. Cinnamon is the sweet, powdered inner bark residue from mighty evergreen trees native to India and China. **Cinnamon essential oils are available, but should not be used internally. Supplements of Cinnamon are available, though it can of course be used in meals or in a tea or tincture at home.**

• Cinnamon effects insulin receptors and helps create glycogen, a storable sugar. Daily use can perhaps help type 2 Diabetics manage their blood sugar levels.

• Studies from both Japan and Canada revealed that Cinnamon also helps lower blood pressure and bad cholesterol in turn.

Avoid consuming large amounts of Cinnamon if you have liver issues. Avoid applying Cinnamon essential oil to the skin, as it may cause a burning rash. Do not take medicinal doses while pregnant.

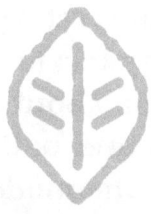

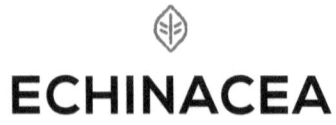

ECHINACEA

(Echinacea spp.)

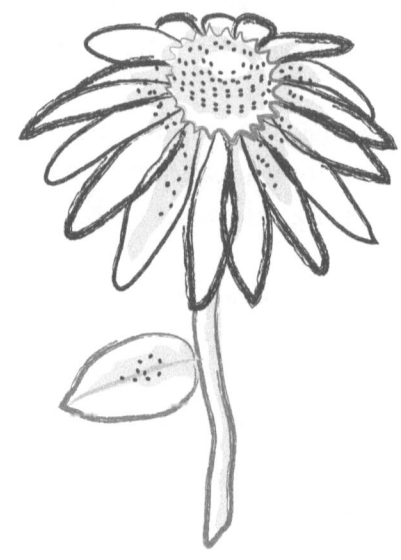

Amazing immunity for colds, flus, and infections

This beautiful prairie flower has received a lot of hype in the herb world for its cold and flu powers. Some treat it like an antibiotic, or even a daily tonic to prevent from getting sick. In truth, Echinacea just empowers the immune system to fight acute infections, but cannot prevent sickness. **Use about a tablespoon of dried leaves, flowers, or roots and boil for one minute for a cold-fighting infusion. Homemade tinctures and freeze-dried herb capsules are a very popular option, too.**

• Use of Echinacea apparently ramps up the abilities of *"macrophages"* or **white blood cells,** as well as interferons to fight both bacterial and viral infections. Taking the herb every two hours over the duration of a cold alone can shorten the amount of time you deal with cold or flu symptoms.

Avoid use of Echinacea if you have an auto-immune disorder. Avoid use of Echinacea also if you take certain pharmaceuticals or birth control pills—check with your doctor. Do not take higher amounts than recommended.

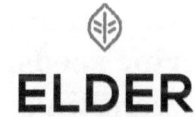

ELDER

(Sambucus nigra)

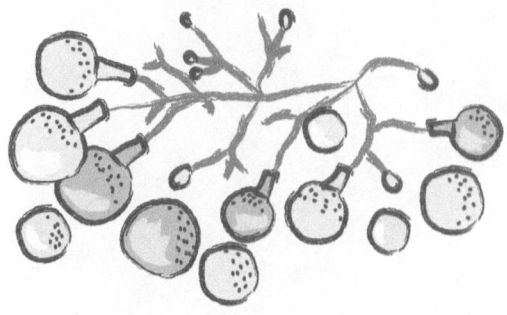

Esteemed virus-fighter and fever supporter of the herb world

If you were to combine Echinacea, Boneset, and Ginger together, you would have an entirely natural herbal medicine to combat any cold or flu that comes your way. Add Elder, however: and all your bases are covered! This vivid, dark purple berry is not only delicious—it also stimulates the immune system and combats viruses. **Dried Elderberries make a delicious tea or infusion, and a tasty tincture. Drink 2-3 cups or take 2-3 droppers a day while sick. Elder supplements are out there, too.**

• Laboratory studies documented Elder extracts acting exactly like antiviral medicine, particularly for combating the flu. Elder might in fact help fight any viral or respiratory infection, like colds, flu, or bronchitis.

• Elder increases the body's ability to produce inflammatory "cytokines" during fevers, which are responsible for killing infections via the immune system.

Do not eat unripe berries or other parts of Elder plant. All parts, including unripe seeds, are slightly toxic and may produce nausea, vomiting, confusion, dizziness, and fainting. Use cautiously if you have an auto-immune condition.

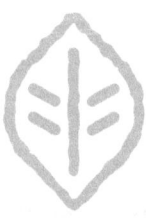

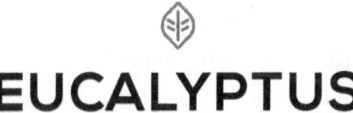

EUCALYPTUS

(Eucalyptus globulus)

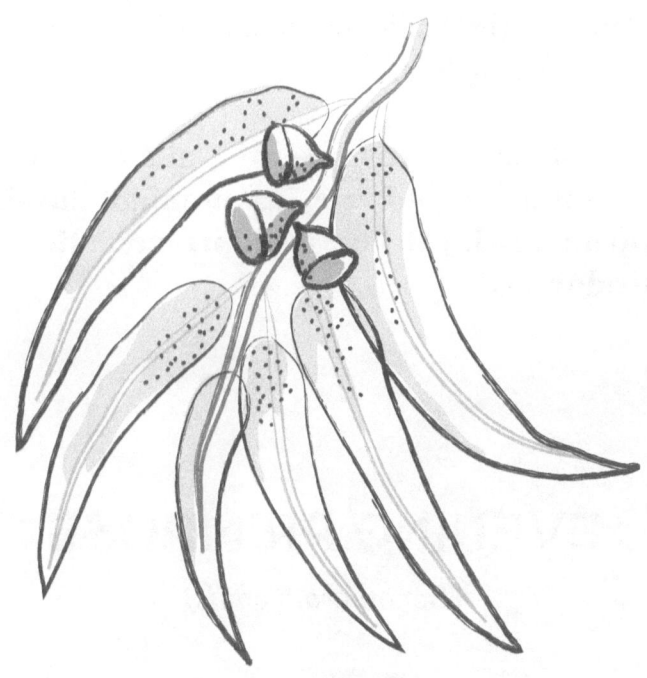

Australia's premier herb for respiratory healing

A stunning Aussie tree now found all over the world, Eucalyptus has snuck its way into many over-the-counter cough medicines—maybe without us realizing we depend on plant healing already! Oils in the leaves are antibacterial, antiviral, and anti-inflammatory, but the plant is especially best at opening up the lungs and assisting with coughs. **Seek out Eucalyptus in essential oils and supplements. Dried leaves are available to make teas, tinctures, salves and oils for healing as well.**

• A volatile oil in Eucalyptus, eucalyptol, acts as an "expectorant" and "bronchiodilator." These actions help open up air passageways, stimulate productive cough, and produce a thinner mucus that can more easily be expelled.

• Eucalyptol is also antibacterial and antiviral, helping kill off illness and infection while also relieving respiratory symptoms. This plant's natural oils are found in many cold-fighting lozenges, syrups, pills, and even chest-rubs.

Do not ingest Eucalyptus essential oils for any reason. Diabetics should avoid use, as it might lower blood sugar. Do not use if you take certain medications. Check with your doctor.

EVENING PRIMROSE

(Oenothera biennis)

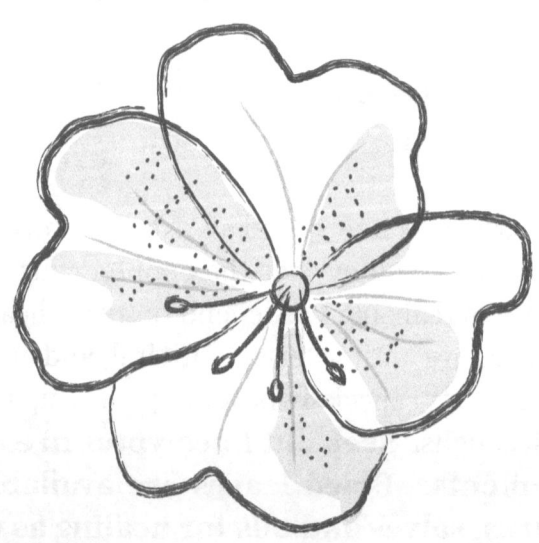

An herbal source for Omega-3's and inflammation soothing

Because it blooms in the evening, Evening Primrose is given a unique, mysterious name. Its benefits are not so mysterious though—high amounts of plant mucilage contain Omega-3 fatty acids, making it a target in the herbal world for dealing with inflammatory issues. **Evening Primrose is active only in oil form—look out for oil capsules or topical oils at natural food stores. If you are an advanced herbalist, try making your own sun-infused oil of the seed pods.**

• Evening Primrose oil (compared to a placebo) helps improve symptoms of inflamed joints in Rheumatoid Arthritis patients, due to Omega-3's ability to modulate inflammation.

• Like Omega-3's found in anything else, Evening Primrose helps lower cholesterol, blood pressure, and the risk for heart disease.

If experiencing discomforts, discontinue use. Avoid excessive use internally if pregnant.

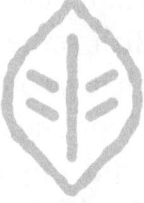

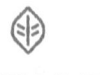

GOLDENSEAL

(Hydrastis canadensis)

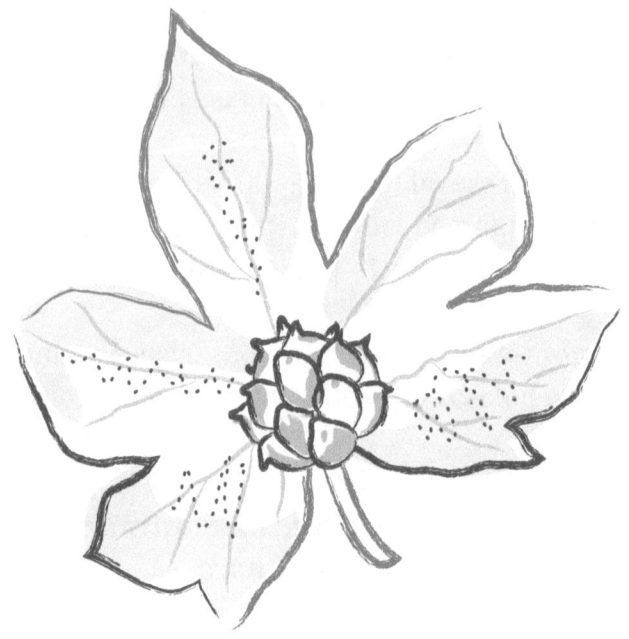

Nature's magic, natural antibiotic and digestive tonic

Goldenseal's use originated among the Native Americans, who then introduced it to English settlers. Today, it has achieved study and reputation enough to be one of the most wildly popular herbs—though it does hold an endangered status. Traditional and mainstream medicine alike uphold it as an antibiotic and healer of numerous digestive issues. **Use the dried root to make a (very bitter) tea, tincture, ointment or salve. Supplements are available—topical use can help with skin infections, internal for digestive ones.**

• Goldenseal's active alkaloid, *berberine,* has proven efficient at combating stomach or intestinal infections like Giardia, E. Coli, amoebic dysentery, or *H. pylori*, bacteria that cause peptic ulcers.

• Topically, *berberine* helps fight fungal infections and alleviate psoriasis. Its powers also enter the arena of the cold-fighting world—Goldenseal's alkaloid also heightens immunity, which can help fight colds (though it cannot kill viruses).

Do not use if pregnant. Check with your doctor before using Goldenseal if you take prescription medications.

MILK THISTLE

(Silybum marianum)

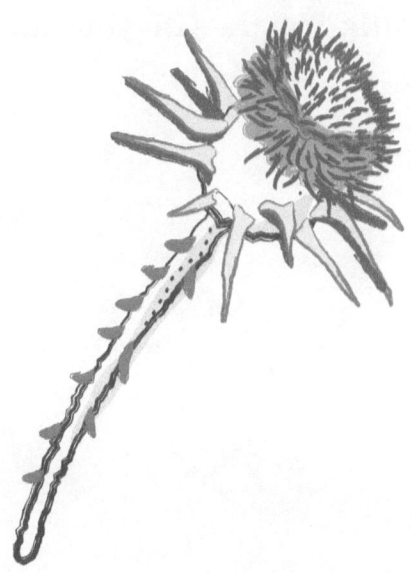

A one-of-a-kind liver herb,
unparalleled in modern medicine

Rarely is there a plant out there that can achieve what mainstream medications cannot. Milk Thistle is the exception. A spiny plant, the seeds nonetheless have unmistakable powers on the liver. It might be just the healer for those experiencing liver issues. **One can make a tea of the seeds as a home remedy. Milk Thistle supplements are readily available at most stores in capsule form.**

• Milk Thistle's healing compound, *silymarin*, prevents toxins and harmful chemicals from literally entering liver cells. It thus protects the liver from damage—even from alcohol, poisons, alkaloids, and NSAID's (like Ibuprofen). Seed preparations are even commonplace in European emergency rooms for mushroom poisoning.

• The same compound catalyzes detoxification in the liver as well, making it a candidate for supporting Hepatitis A, B, C, Cirrhosis, and Jaundice.

Discuss use of Milk Thistle with your doctor if you have liver issues.

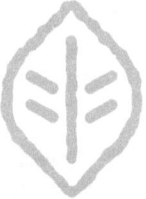

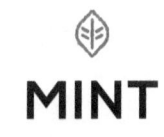

MINT

(Mentha spp.)

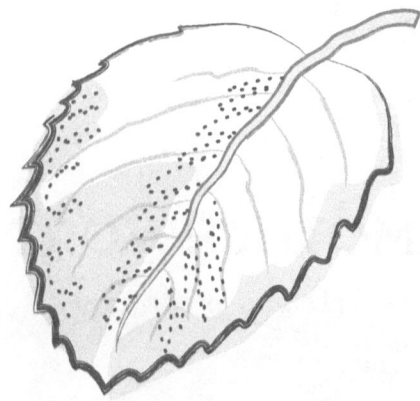

A cooling, soothing must-have herb for mind and body

Who could forget Mint? One of the most popular herbs, Spearmint and Peppermint alike are well-used and documented for their calming effects, not just on the nerves and mind—but also on the digestive tract, and for coughs, colds, and flus. **Making a tea at home for use every day is perfectly safe, and Mints make excellent, tasty tinctures. Also seek Mints in cough crops, syrups, capsules, and essential oil form.**

• Peppermint/Spearmint's active compounds soothe cramps, pain, indigestion, and flatulence in the digestive tract. In the meantime, they also help calm the mind.

• Topical applications of essential oils help with nervous pains and aches, even headaches.

• Menthol in all mints has found its way into many a cough and cold remedy. It acts as a decongestant, opens airways, soothes coughs, and expels mucus.

Do not apply essential oils to infants or small children. Avoid using Peppermint if you have heartburn, GERD or a hernia.

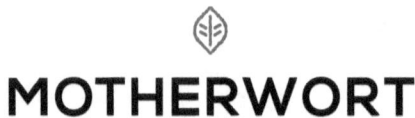

MOTHERWORT

(Leonurus cardiac)

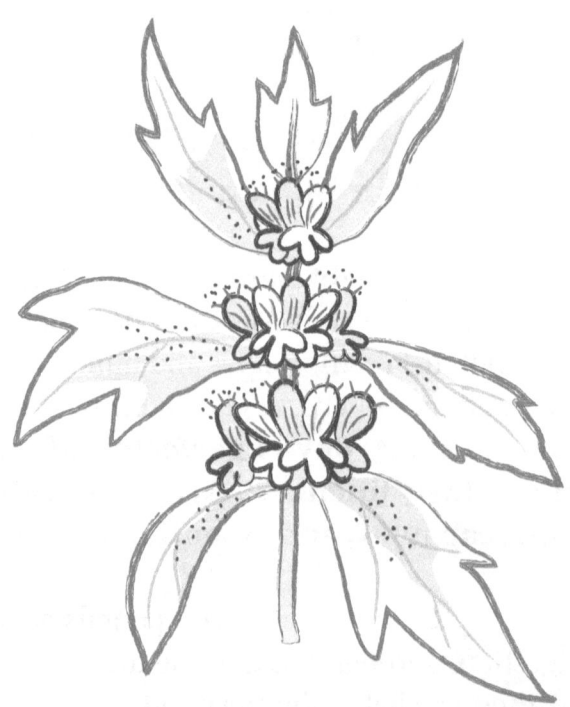

A heart-warming ally for cardiovascular health

Some may plague Motherwort as a noxious weed, with spiny,

irritating burrs that attach to your clothes. Little do they know: a preparation of leaves and flowers could be one of the most astounding natural heart tonics out there! **Make and use your own homemade tea or tincture, if you desire. Motherwort supplements are not uncommon either, and are an option at natural food grocers.**

• A Chinese study observed Motherwort relaxing cells in the heart muscle. This then modulated blood pressure, strengthened heartbeat, and even showed the ability to regulate certain heart arrhythmias or palpitations.

• The same heart effects have an ability to reduce anxiety, tension, and nervousness.

People taking clotting medications or with clotting disorders should avoid Motherwort. Avoid use too if you are pregnant.

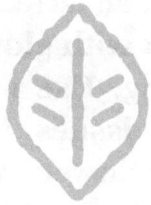

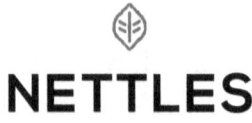

NETTLES

(Urtica dioica)

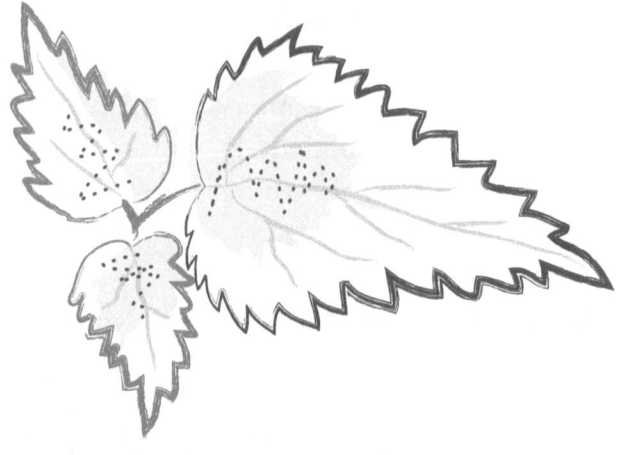

A stinging plant, overlooked superfood, and inflammation healer

Did you know Stinging Nettles are more nutritious than any plants that might grow in your garden? That includes Kale, Spinach, and Lettuce. Think twice next time you pull on gloves to remove them like a weed. Keeping those non-flowering, seedless Nettle tops might make for an incredibly nutritious supplement or relief for allergies. **Pick with gloves, hang, and dry for 1 hour to remove the sting. Use a tincture or supplement for allergy and urinary issues, or cook up greens from Nettle tops before they flower. Opt for a thick infusion of the leaves for Nettle's nutritional content, excellent for the anemic or undernourished.**

• Nettles are a significant source of Vitamins A, B6, and C, Antioxidants, Protein, Potassium, Magnesium, Manganese, Iron and Phosphorus.

• Nettles suppress histamine response—great for allergy relief. A noted diuretic, this can be cleansing for urinary health. Studies even demonstrate an ability to reduce prostate growth in men.

Avoid use if you are pregnant. Avoid long-term use as well with diuretic herbs—they deplete potassium stores and lead to electrolyte imbalance.

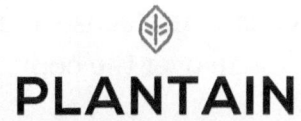

PLANTAIN

(Plantago spp.)

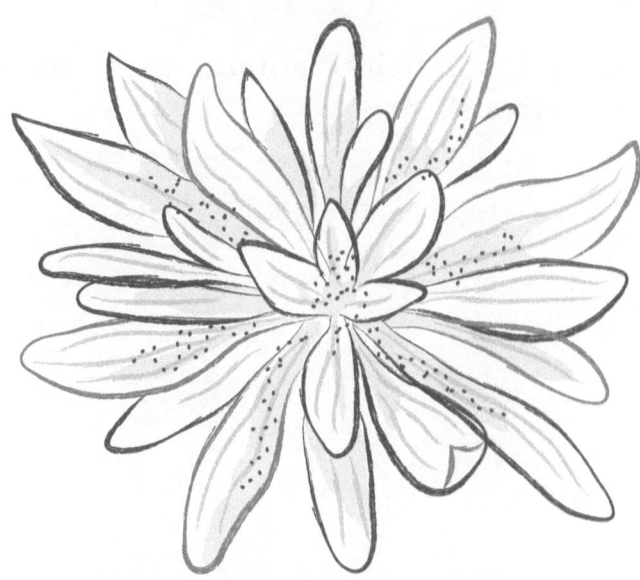

Not a banana - but a beneficial, understated stomach healer

Plantain is a ubiquitous herb, found practically everywhere in the world. Once upon a time it was revered as a cleansing, cancer-fighting folk remedy—there's no evidence of that, but today it instead holds the trophy as a digestive tonic, laxative, and topical wound healer. **Incorporate Plantain into oils and salves for topical use, or consider a piping hot tea for bowel irregularity.**

• One Plantain species, "Psyllium," has seeds that are popular, over-the-counter remedies for constipation. They certainly work—all Plantains have laxative action, so give it a try.

• The leaves are high in fiber and Omega-3's. Raw Plantain leaves added to salads can cleanse the digestive tract, and improve inflammation all over the body.

• Chew up and poultice Plantain leaves on itchy skin, rashes, bug bites and stings. It provides immediate relief!

Avoid eating too much Plantain, as it may create excessive laxative effect.

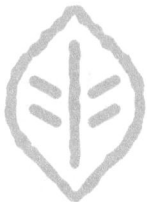

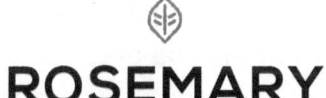

ROSEMARY

(Rosmarinus officinalis)

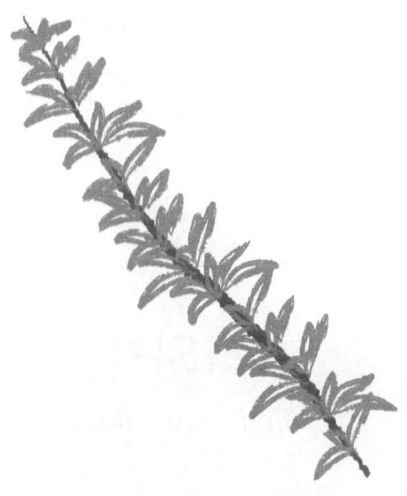

A mind-enhancing, anti-oxidant rich, delicious spice

Rosemary is probably more well-known for perking up roasted vegetables and Mediterranean dishes. But its history of addition to foods is not only for taste—its antioxidant capabilities were so powerful they prevented foods from oxidizing and going rancid. Those same antioxidant capabilities can be amazing for age-fighting, while other compounds can kill bacteria, improve circulation, and reduce inflammation. **Essential oils and supplements are common, though you can add a sprig to boiling water for tea, or craft a D.I.Y. tincture.**

• Rosemary's powers to improve circulation are noted for helping stimulate and clarify mental function over time. Coupled with its antioxidants, this makes Rosemary and excellent supplement for the elderly.

• The same circulation-enhancing help open up air passage-ways, assisting with breathing and working as a decongestant for coughs or colds. Rosemary's antimicrobial could also be a further boon for combating infection of illnesses themselves.

Medicinal doses of Rosemary are not recommended during pregnancy. Do not ingest essential oil, and discontinue use if it causes burns on skin.

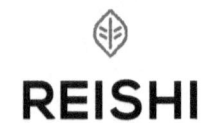

REISHI

(Ganoderma tsugae)

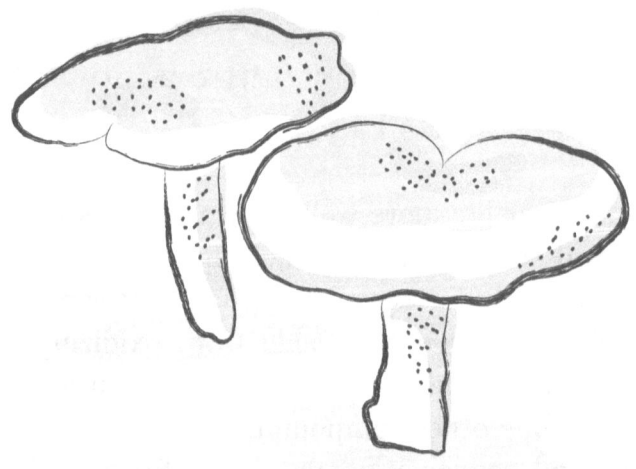

An immune-boosting mushroom for allergies and inflammation

Most wouldn't think of mushrooms as being medicinal, yet modern research is quickly proving that they are. At the front of this research is Reishi, an enormously gorgeous fungus with species native to both Asia and North America. Adaptogenic, anti-inflammatory, and even anti-tumor effects have been noted. **You can use it in a tea, tincture, or extract at home, though most find its taste terribly bitter. Supplements are widely available at natural food stores.**

• Reishi contains polysaccharides and triterpenes, which modulate the immune system's creation of inflammation. It can thus help with the pain and management of auto-immune disorders—like Rheumatoid Arthritis or Lupus.

• These same immune benefits can help with chronic allergies over time, whether sinus, respiratory, or even food-related allergies or sensitivities.

Avoid using Reishi if you take blood pressure medication or anti-coagulant drugs. Stop use altogether if you develop allergy symptoms.

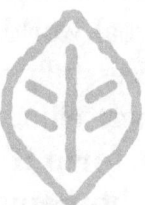

ST. JOHN'S WORT

(Hypericum perforatum)

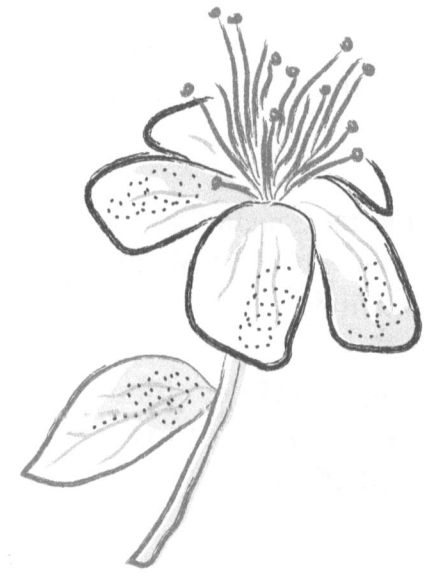

Combat depression and melancholy
- naturally and effectively

This bright yellow, populous flower is practically synonymous with depression in the herbal world. Anciently and modernly, St. John's Wort is used successfully for minor depression issues, and might be one of the bestselling herbs of today. **Try it in tincture or supplement form if you've got the blues. It makes a lovely tea and homemade extract, as well as a gorgeous, deep-red salve or oil.**

• Trials with St. John's Wort proved that it was more effective than a placebo, and just as effective as mainstream mediations for mild to moderate depressions and anxiety. It's active ingredient, *hypericin,* acts quite a bit like an MAOI inhibiter.

• Not many may know that beyond depression, St. John's Wort is a very functional topical nerve pain-reliever. Salves or oils are rubbed into the skin for pain relief.

Do not take St. John's Wort if you use other prescription medications—the plant enhances liver clearance and can nullify their effects. The plant also may increase photosensitivity if taken in high amounts over time.

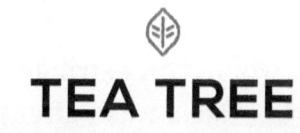

TEA TREE

(Melaleuca alternifolia)

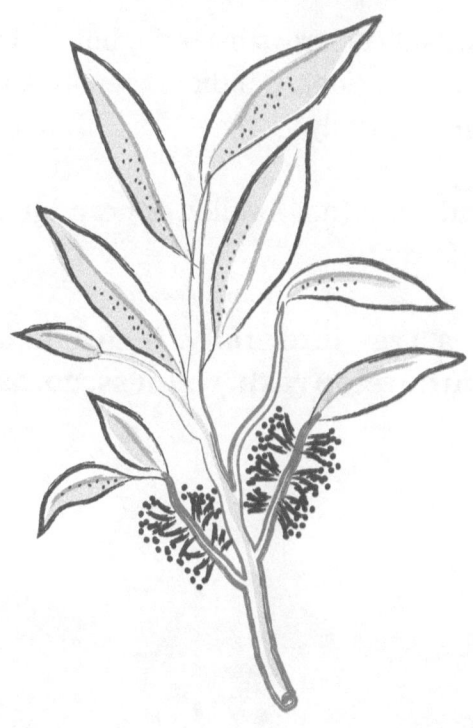

The herbal world's skin healer,
cleanser, and protector

Among herbs, Tea Tree's power as an antimicrobial is almost unrivaled. Originating from Australia (like Eucalyptus), it is now a standard herbal product available everywhere, especially for skin issues and wounds. **It is almost exclusively found only in essential oil form, as its use is exclusively topical, not internal.**

• When applied to the skin, Tea Tree can rid you of any infection imaginable. Oils in the plant have been observed destroying and inhibiting *Staphylococcus* bacteria, even antibiotic-resistant strains. Use it as a wound cleanser in a pinch.

• Tea Tree makes a wonderful astringent for acne, as it kills acne-causing bacteria. Use a wash after poison ivy, sumac, or oak exposure to prevent outbreak.

• Tea Tree not only destroys bacteria, but fungus as well. Use it also for Athlete's Foot, Candida, toenail, and vaginal yeast infections, only topically.

• A gargle and rinse (not swallowed) can kill mouth bacteria and prevent gingivitis.

Never take Tea Tree internally, it can be fatal. Discontinue use if you develop rash, redness, contact dermatitis or allergy.

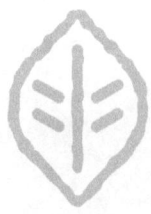

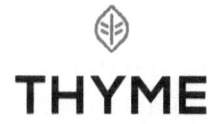

THYME

(Thymus vulgaris)

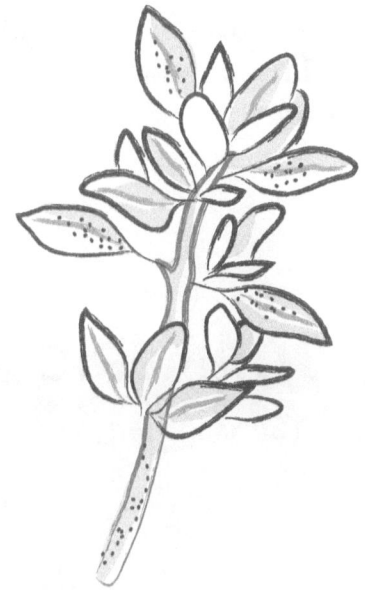

A sprig of flavor for the cough, cold, and respiratory spells

Much like Eucalyptus and Mint, Thyme too has snuck its way into many an over-the-counter cold and flu remedy. This is probably because this culinary herb also has bronchio-dilating, deconges- tant, expectorant, and anti-microbial powers. **Make a tea of the sprigs, or keep your own tincture for use at home. It's also found as a popular essential oil for topical use, and healing supplement for internal use.**

• Thyme's properties act through thymol, a volatile oil that helps open up the airways and clear mucus. At the same time it helps inhibit the growth of viruses that causes colds and flus— probably the reason why *thymol* is also found in commercial cough syrups and lozenges.

• *Thymol* is also the anti-microbial ingredient in some mouth-washes. Consider using Thyme as a mouth rinse for preventing gingivitis and mouth infections.

Do not use Thyme essential oil internally. Consult your doctor if you are taking medicinal doses of Thyme and you have thyroid issues.

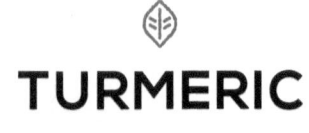

TURMERIC

(Curcuma longa)

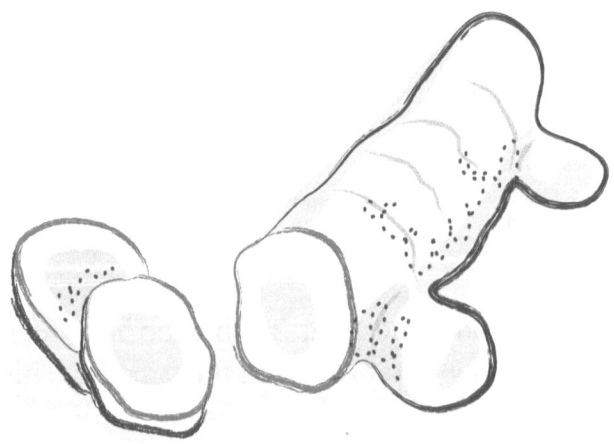

A curry cornerstone that heals digestive inflammation

Yes, Turmeric is most famous for adding color, body, and deep flavor to curry blends from India. But in the country's culinary and Ayurvedic traditions, the bright yellow powdered root miraculously soothed inflammation like no other. Today, its properties are highly celebrated, respected, and touted all over the world by science and tradition alike. **Oils and salves make excellent topical anti-inflammatories, though temporarily dye your hands yellow. Feel free to make your own homemade teas or tinctures—or take an easy-to-find supplement from your store.**

• Turmeric's active ingredient, curcumin, is an anti-inflammatory especially influential on the digestive tract. Research shows that it eases the symptoms of those with Crohn's Disease, IBS (Irritable Bowel Syndrome), and Colitis.

• Topical applications have also been seeing helping the inflammatory pain of Rheumatoid and Osteo-arthritis alike.

Avoid taking excessively large amounts. Avoid using Turmeric if you have a blood clotting disorder or take blood clotting medication.

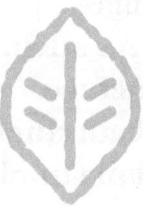

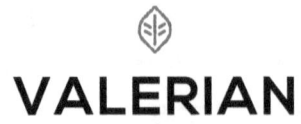

VALERIAN

(Valeriana officinalis)

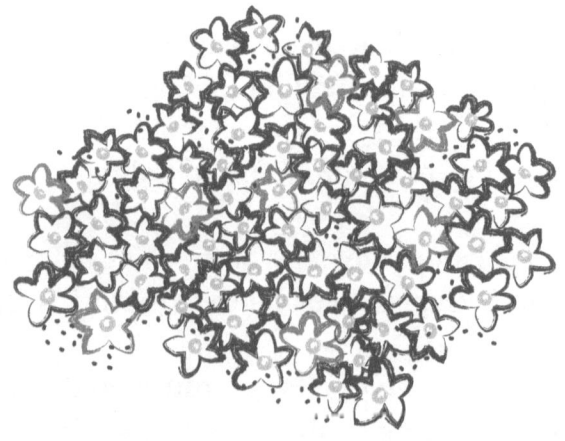

An herbal lullaby to dispel insomnia, or soothe anxiety

Valerian has quite the reputation. Not only is it synonymous with "sleep aid" in the herbal world, most should be aware that the compounds found in Valerian are also responsible for the qualities found in Valium—a prescription drug that slightly echoes the plant's name. **As such, be cautious using it as a homemade tea or tincture. Drink only 1 cup of tea before bed per day, and cut tincture dosage in half. One can easily obtain Valerian supplements and tinctures at natural grocers.**

• Many studies demonstrate Valerian's ability to improve sleep without creating any morning fog. Its active constituents, *valerenic acid* and *valerenol*, bind to receptors in the brain that promote relaxation and sleepiness—the same receptors that mainstream drugs might target.

• Valerian can help untangle restlessness for a single night of sleep in someone expecting giddiness the next day. For those with long-term insomnia problems, Valerian tends to work better with other calming herbs like Lemon Balm or even Hops *(Humulus lupus)* and used for 1-2 two weeks every day.

Avoid taking herb in unusually high amounts, which can cause uncomfortable symptoms like dizziness, giddiness, and nausea. Stop use if you experience immediate giddiness—Valerian has a stimulating, anxiety-increasing influence on about 10% of the population.

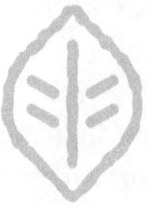

CHAPTER 4

Most Common Maladies and their Herbal Preventives

In our previous chapters, I armed you with my *30 Top Favorite* herbs for combating minor illnesses and ailments at home. *Five* of them I consider my front-line allies and herbal protectors, which you can review in Chapter 2.

Chapter 3, on the other hand, provided you with information and healing capabilities of yet more: *25 additional botanical remedies for further illness and injury-fighting, in a pinch!* **Using all these plants together, supported by research and traditional herbalism hand-in-hand, there is no single malady or sickness that you won't be equipped to face at home; whether alone, or with family or loved ones.**

It might be confusing at first figuring out how to navigate which ones to use, when, and for what. That's what this following section is for.

Use this chapter as a reference guide, compass, and organized manual to help you decide which herbs to use for your specific condition—which ones work best compared to others, as well as their more minor nuances. **Make sure that you also cross-reference each individual herb's entry as it is listed in previous chapters for the most well-rounded, complete approach on how to use it, and when it's best to use it!**

Remember too: if you feel you are developing a chronic illness, dangerous infection, or other serious medical condition, *please do not rely on the use of herbs.* Visit your doctor or the emergency room, when in doubt—but for the minor scraps, colds and skin problems at home, you can safely turn to herbs for the following *Common Maladies.*

Nervous Conditions

Whether we want to admit it or not, our nerves and brains are often one of the primary determining aspects of our health that relay a sense of well-being. Our bodies might be in tip-top shape—but if our nerves are frayed, or our mood depressed, we must start with healing our minds first and then working our way outward.

In the arena of nervous conditions, herbal remedies truly shine. There are a myriad of herbs that do well to calm our spirits, as well as nervous conditions they help smooth over. Reference the following herbs for your nerves:

Headaches

Headaches are annoying and life-hampering. They can have a wide variety of causes, too. Consider some herbal methods below for more commonplace, minor sinus headaches.

• **Ginger** – This especially comes in handy for allergy, sinus-headaches with lots of inflammation. Eat a meal with lots of Ginger, sip a Ginger ale, or enjoy some hot Chai tea (which contains Ginger). Or, make yourself some hot Ginger root tea.

• **Eucalyptus** – Dab just a bit of essential oil, only one drop each, on the sides of your temples.

• **Lemon Balm** – For nervous, anxiety, or digestive-related headaches, try some hot Lemon Balm tea from the fresh bruised leaves.

Stress and Anxiety

No one likes to feel stressed out or uptight. Some among us deal with stress and anxiety as a part of our daily routine, or even as symptoms of larger diagnosed nervous disorders that can disrupt well-being. Maybe try some of the following remedies:

• **Alfalfa** – Provides nutrition for those so nervous and stressed out, that it interferes with eating habits. Eat leaves or sprouts raw, or in a hot infusion over long term.

• **Ashwagandha** – Like Alfalfa, is a nutritive tonic for digestion wrecked by anxiety and nerves. Roots and berries in a hot infusion daily, or a fixed syrup, over the long term.

• **Lemon Balm** – Helps calm acute instances of nervousness or anxiety. Helps whether in tea or tincture form, as long as the herb is fresh.

• **Nettles** – Nutritive qualities strengthen those weak from stress or adrenal fatigue. Fresh or dried leaves from non-flowering plant tops in a thick infusion every day, or cooked as greens over the long term.

Depression

Minor to moderate depression can be supported by the use of herbs. However, if you suffer from severe clinical depression, please turn to the guidance of your doctor and counselor. Otherwise, think about using these for your troubles:

• **Lemon Balm** – Can help with mild depressions, tastes great and very calming. Use as tea, tincture, or sometimes supplement daily for the long term.

• **St. John's Wort** – Proven to help with mild to moderate depressions. Consider combining with Lemon Balm. Most commonly comes as tincture or supplement used daily for the long term.

Sleep

Sleep disturbance can be the result of other nervous conditions. You might be wound up tight with anxiety, or heavy with thoughts from depression, with sleep always just out of reach. Try these herbs that classically bring you calm, peaceful dreams.

• **Lemon Balm** – Take tincture or a hot tea of this fresh herb ½ to 1 hour before bed. It might soothe not only depression or anxiety, but get you some rest.

• **Valerian** – For really wound-up, mind-racing nights, Valerian does the trick—often with more power than Lemon Balm. However, try the two together to increase your chances: they are a common blend. Tea, tincture, or supplement work great.

Infections

Before modern antibiotics, herbs were used traditionally all over the world to heal infected wounds of all kinds. Whether bacterial, fungal, or viral, there would be some herb that could do the trick;

sometimes there were powerful herbs that could take care of all three kinds of infection!

Even today, antibiotics sometimes fall short of fighting an infection. Numerous antibiotic-resistant bacterial strains are out there, which don't respond to modern drugs. Viruses and fungi often leave us helpless too, since antibiotics simply don't have an effect.

Someday, we might find ourselves turning to herbs for the following maladies, as they give us an infinitely variable chemical retaliation against bacteria, viruses, and fungi alike!

Wounds and Cuts

Some herbs are way more antiseptic than we give them credit for. Even better, we might have them in the kitchen or garden when we didn't even realize it! Some of the following are good examples to use for minor cuts and scrapes:

• **Comfrey** – On very minor, superficial cuts, Comfrey kills germs and speeds healing and closure. ***Do not*** use in salve or oil form—rather, make a tea or infusion, or use store-bought or homemade tincture as a wound wash. You may poultice the leaves or root straight on the wound too, and wash away later.

• **Plantain** – Similar to Comfrey, Plantain helps disinfect very small, minor cuts or scrapes. Healing accelerates as well. Tea or infusion as a wound wash works well, but a poultice of the chewed up leaves and seeds works wonders.

• **Tea Tree** – For deeper, more worrisome wounds, use a Tea Tree tincture, liniment, or tea as a wound wash. Try diluting 5 drops essential oil in a cup of water as a wash also. ***Never apply undiluted essential oils straight on a wound. Please go immediately to the emergency room for*** *major wounds.*

Pink Eye

It's rarely a huge worry. But nonetheless, pink eye (also called "conjunctivitis") is an irritating, annoying infection that can keep you home from work for days—or keep your kids from school when they are otherwise absolutely fine. Try these home remedies though, and see if they can cut down on infection time.

• **Rosemary** – Make a strong tea or infusion, well strained and cooled, and use it as an eye wash 3 times per day.

• **Spearmint** – Similar to Rosemary, make a strong tea or infusion of this fragrant plant and rinse the eyes 3 times per day. Make sure it is strained and cooled.

Ear Ache and Infection

These kind of infections might be the side effect of a cold, flu, or sinus infection. They are annoying all the same—especially in little ones! The following is an herbal remedy commonly used for ear aches and infections:

• **Garlic** – Chop up 1 to 5 cloves of Garlic, and heat on the stove very low in a bit of olive oil in a saucepan. After 10 minutes, strain Garlic from the oil. Add about 5 drops to infected, pained ear. Tilt head or cover with a cotton ball for another 10 minutes.

Coughs, Colds and Flu

These most common of maladies can be healed and assisted by the most common of herbs. Next time you or a loved one catch cold, try these out to see if they cut down on the duration of your illness. Science says they could work!

• **Boneset** – Make a hot infusion of the dried leaves, or take a dried leaf tincture 3 times every day for the duration of your cold or flu—especially if you are experiencing symptoms of fever.

• **Echinacea** – Make several cups of hot infusion from the leaves, flowers, and roots to be taken every 2 hours while sick. Or, opt for a dose of Echinacea tincture or capsule every 2 hours.

• **Elder** – Boil or simmer a Tbsp. of dried, ripe berries in water for colds or flus with fever. A cold-steeped juice is very medicinal as well, packed with Vitamin C. Take tea, tincture, or supplement freely throughout the duration of your illness.

• **Garlic** – Crush, chop, chew (yes, chew), then immediately swallow up to 10 cloves of Garlic per day while you have a cold or flu. Try following each clove with a glass of plant-based milk like almond, rice, or soy. During the length of your cold, you might find that loved ones do not want to come near you. Garlic teas or tinctures won't do you much good!

Fungal Infections

These happen more often than you might think. The most common brush-ins with fungal infections include Athlete's Foot and some skin afflictions, and then there is the dreaded yeast infection among women. Looking for a more natural solution? The following herbs are well-known fungus-fighters.

• **Garlic** – Poultice Garlic straight on your skin for dermal fungal infections (it will sting). Traditionally, Garlic cloves were crushed and inserted straight into the vaginal canal for yeast infections. It might be a bit strange and feel unusual—but scientifically, it should work, if you're bold.

• **Goldenseal** – Infuse the root in a tea or tincture, and apply topically for dermal fungal infections, like Athlete's Foot. Berberine's qualities tend to do the trick. You can also find Goldenseal creams or ointments at some stores.

• **Tea Tree** – This herb is priority for Athlete's Foot and yeast infections alike. Add a few drops of essential oil to water as a wash or douche for either.

Immunity

When it comes to health, focusing on our Immune Systems is something that often gets passed up. It is, however, at the root of many issues, interestingly enough.

In modern medicine beliefs, a lot of times instead of strengthening our Immune Systems, we lose sight of what's truly wrong. We might try to treat separate symptoms related exclusively to a sickness, instead of looking deeper at the underlying problem, for example.

As we strive to find relief for yet more minute and detailed symptoms, we get farther and farther away from the bigger picture: immunity! The following illnesses or symptoms are great examples that are in fact warning signs that we are straying from a strong immune system.

Allergies

This relates to sinus allergies, such as to seasonal pollen or pet dander; or to minor food intolerances or hypersensitivities, like with gluten or dairy. If you experience those symptoms or troubles, it might be that your immune system needs a little kick. *Full blown food allergies, such as to peanuts and shellfish, are a different matter—please rely on mainstream medicine to treat or allay life-threatening allergies.*

• **Ginger** – Taking this pungent, hot root will not only rev up your immune system. It can also help soothe inflammation of the sinuses or digestive tract that are worked up by allergens. Take it every day for a few months in a tea or tincture form, 2-3 times per day, to feel its effects.

• **Nettles** – Nettles might be a more short-term remedy for allergies, and only of the nasal kind. Tea, tincture, or freeze-dried herb capsules act somewhat like an antihistamine. On long-term basis it can boost the immune system, especially in the wake of adrenal fatigue due to nourishing vitamins and minerals.

• **Reishi** – A premier "adaptogen," Reishi is powerful for the immune system and helps it adapt better responses to all sorts of allergens—airborne or food-related. Take it long term: in capsule form works best. If you are daring, try making a bitter but medicinal tea or tincture and taking that daily for several weeks.

Fevers

Many treat fevers as a dangerous, worrisome part of the cold or flu experience. But really, fevers are a healthy sign—it means that your immune system is working. Fevers are produced by the immune system to kill viruses, bacteria, and expel waste or foreign invaders through the lungs and skin (through sweat). Rather than stifling a fever: support your fever! These herbs can help.

• **Boneset** – Before modern medicine, Boneset was relied on to combat Dengue fever and Malaria, two dangerous febrile conditions. Use the dried leaves of this plant in a hot infusion, 2-3 times a day, while sick with cold or flu with fever.

• **Elder** – Elder has been observed supporting the body's own fever conditions, which produce inflammation to kill bacteria or viruses. Make hot infusions of ripe Elderberry tea, and drink freely while experiencing feverish symptoms.

Energy and Longevity

The greatest herbs for the immune system are often called "adaptogens" or "tonics." Some of these can be considered adaptogens, while others might not quite hold that definition. Either way, these are all known to amplify immunity, and not only help better deal with allergies or sickness—but to increase energy, livelihood, well-being, and even longevity!

• **Alfalfa** – Chock full of vitamins and minerals (including Vitamin K, Iron, and Zinc), Alfalfa not only nourishes: it brings energy, strong immunity, and even cancer prevention to the table. Add it raw as sprouts/leaves to salads and meals, or take a hot, thick infusion every day.

• **Ashwagandha** – The roots and berries in a nourishing infusion every day contain iron and magnesium, as well as antioxidants that help the body cope and revitalize in the face of stress. It has helped many regain energy, especially in recovering sexual health and libido.

• **Reishi** – Taking Reishi daily enriches the body with polysaccharides and triterpenes, compounds that help the immune system modulate itself in the healthiest way possible. Hence, it protects against cancers and auto-immune issues. Take it in capsule form, or a bitter, homemade tea or tincture.

Digestive Issues

Issues with gut health are easily the most common problems we deal with. Traditional herbalists have found more than enough plant-based responses to the discomforts, pains, and unpleasant bowel habits that can form from diminished digestive health. Luckily enough too, modern research and evidence joins hands with traditional knowledge to provide more than enough herbal solutions to tummy aches and belly upsets. Explore the following, if you're wanting a break from modern meds.

Stomach Aches and Cramps

These things happen. Whether or not it's due to something you ate—or accompanied with unpleasant, stinky aftermath—some herbs can smooth out the kinks in your tummy. Here are my top choices.

• **Lemon Balm** – This nerve-calming herb also curbs jitters in your stomach. Whether its cramps, aches, gas, or "butterflies," try a cup of hot Lemon Balm tea or a bit of tincture. Take a bit more each half hour until symptoms go away.

• **Mint** – Similarly to Lemon Balm, Mint's effects are surprisingly quick and noticeable for belly troubles. "After-dinner mints" did originate from the occasional need to allay flatulence or aches after meals. Chew on a fresh leaf, make a warm tea, or try tincture.

Nausea

Arguably the most upsetting digestive symptom out there, a few herbs can be spectacular at curbing nausea. Compared to modern pills and other remedies for nausea, the simple use of some fairly easy to find plants can be much more appealing.

• **Ginger** – This root is famous for its anti-nausea miracles. Chew on the root, make tea, or even sip Ginger ale with real Ginger in it. You'll feel the effects!

• **Thyme** – Like Ginger, Thyme works surprisingly will for nausea issues. In traditional medicine, it was used to ease morning nausea in pregnant women. If you can't get a hand on some Ginger, try out Thyme instead—nibble on a few leaves, or make a tea from the sprigs.

Constipation

When you haven't "gone" for a day or two, and it's getting uncomfortable, a few herbs might be able to help you get going. Try the following selections out. If you experience constipation for longer than a week, however, check in with your doctor and don't depend exclusively on herbs.

• **Plantain** – Take several leaves and seeds from this easy-to-find plant, chop them up, and steep them in cold water for a day. If you like—set the sun-tea on the windowsill for a day to help gently extract the plant's mucilage. Drink 2 times a day until you see improvement. *Also:* try adding leaves to a smoothie or juice blend.

• **Aloe Vera** – Aloe juice, which is easy to find at grocery stores, is purported to have a mild laxative effect and detoxifying influence on the gut. Try some Aloe juice—but avoid taking Aloe leaf, gel, or other parts internally for constipation. The painful side effects are unpleasant, and often not worth the trouble.

Diarrhea

Opposite of constipation, diarrhea makes for another unpleasant digestive reality. Luckily, most cases of diarrhea are incredibly easy to support and treat with herbs. If you experience chronic diarrhea for longer than a week, however, check in with your doctor—especially if herbs aren't helping. It could be dangerous not to.

• **Goldenseal** – If you are worried that your diarrhea is caused by amoebic dysentery, parasites, food poisoning, or digestive infection, Goldenseal will save the day. Keep in mind: this plant will help destroy the diarrhea-causing infection, but not alleviate the diarrhea itself. Take it as a tea, tincture, or supplement.

• **Plantain** – This plant happens to be good for both constipation and diarrhea. Take several leaves and seeds, chop them up, and steep them in cold water for a day—or add them to a smoothie or juice. If you like—set the sun-tea on the windowsill for a day to help gently extract the plant's mucilage. Drink 2 times a day until you see improvement.

Aches and Pains

Did you know that our modern day sources of certain pain-relieving drugs—like Aspirin, for example—originated from plants? That is something to consider, especially when reaching out for more natural options for pain relief.

Arthritis

So many herbs out there tout anti-inflammatory capabilities. If you have pains from arthritis, whether Rheumatoid or Osteo-arthritis, there is an immense selection from the world of herbs to choose from. In fact—almost *all* herbs have some sort of anti-inflammatory capability! However, try out and stick to the following: they have the most supported use, both in modern studies and traditional knowledge.

• **Evening Primrose** – The seed pods are high in Omega-3's, ALA, and GLA. An oil bought commercially, or infused from the plant's seed pods, has been shown to alleviate inflamed joints—especially for Rheumatoid Arthritis sufferers.

• **Arnica** – Creams, ointments, and salves are widely available for arthritis relief at most natural food stores. You can also opt to make your own salve or topical oil by extracting Arnica's soothing compounds from the flowers. *Make sure to not use Arnica internally, only externally on pained joints.*

• **Comfrey** – Comfrey can take the edge off arthritic pain. Creams and ointments are available at some stores—or make an oil or salve from the leaves or root to rub into painful joints. *Do not take internally.*

• **Ginger** – Taken internally, Ginger can help with inflammatory pain much like a modern NSAID (like Acetaminophen). You might need to take it periodically over a few hours—make a fresh Ginger root tea, a Chai tea, or add fresh Ginger to your meal. Or—sip a Ginger ale.

• **Turmeric** – This bright yellow powder can provide relief for arthritis more effectively than any other. Take it internally in a tea, tincture, supplement, or added to food. Or, make yourself a Turmeric oil or salve—it works, but might make your hands yellow for a while!

Pain Relief

What about general pain? Beyond achy joints from arthritis, there are numerous ways we experience pain. For example: we might suffer from muscle pains due to exercise or injury. Or, we might face nerve pain from issues like sciatica, or even type 2 diabetes. No matter the issue, the herbal world will probably have you covered. If you're tiring from pain medications or ointments with uncomfortable side effects—or maybe you just want to make your own remedy, or turn to something natural—check out these herbs which have been used for ages to soothe pains of all kinds.

• **Aloe** – The pain of burns, itching, dry skin, psoriasis, and eczema is no fun. Apply Aloe gel or cream to skin infections, afflictions, or even wounds. It can dull the burn of inflamed pain, and speed up the time it takes to heal.

• **Arnica** – Arnica assuages not only joint pain, but muscle or bruise pains too. Creams, ointments, and salves are commercially available. You can make your own salve or oil from the flowers. ***Do not use internally or on open skin.***

• **Black Haw** – Containing a compound called *scopoletin* (as well as Aspirin-like compounds, including *salicin*), taking the twigs or root of this plant in a hot tea could achieve similar effect as taking Aspirin for tummy aches, menstrual cramps, or even the pain from harsh, dry coughs.

• **Cayenne** – Try an over-the-counter cream containing *capsaicin*, the active ingredient in Cayenne that makes it "spicy." It works excellent on unbroken, smooth skin for nerve and muscle pains especially. Just make sure you wash your hands after using—getting any residue in your eyes or mouth will burn!

• **Comfrey** – Comfrey eases muscle and joint pain both, but also helps speed healing of muscles, breaks, and internal injuries. Make an oil or salve from the leaves or root and rub into skin. ***Do not take internally or on open skin.***

• **St. John's Wort** – Got the blues and some uncomfortable nerve pain? St. John's Wort not only allays depression. When used as a topical oil or salve rubbed into skin, it can soothe nerve pain. Try it with issues like **fibromyalgia**.

Toothache

Maybe you don't have to go to the dentist for simple tooth pain. Instead, turn to the culinary spices and herbs in your kitchen cupboard. If you don't think it's a cavity, abscess, or infection— consider these herbs for ridding yourself of the agony.

• **Echinacea** – Beyond fighting colds, Echinacea was traditionally used for toothaches. Make an oil or salve from leaves, flowers, or roots— apply just a bit to the gums around your aching tooth. Apply more every hour until pain recedes.

• **St. John's Wort** – This plant, typically used for depression, yields a gorgeously deep-red infused oil if you leave it in oil in the sun. It can be safely dabbed around the gums of a throbbing tooth. Apply more every hour until pain recedes.

Sore Throat

Ah—the scratchy, raspy pain that accompanies colds, flu, or sometimes even strep throat or allergies. Luckily, herbal remedies have been in place for sore throats for hundreds of years... if not thousands. All it takes is making a hot, soothing tea with any of the following herbs—and add a little lemon or honey *(a mixture of maple syrup and malt syrup works the same way as a vegan alternative)* for additional throat-relieving effects.

• **Eucalyptus** – This Australian tree's active constituent, *eucalyptol*, helps soothe the pain and soreness of coughs or sore throat. It may also help open up airways, assist breathing, and even kill of viral or bacterial infections causing the sore throat. Make it as a gargle, using a few drops of essential oils or dried leaves. Spit it out when finished.

• **Garlic** – Garlic, like Eucalyptus, is strong at fighting off viral/ bacterial infection causing sore throat. It also boosts immunity to give an added edge. Most of all—a warm Garlic tea can be throat-soothing. Add a few cloves (as many as you can stand) to warm or hot water, then crush them in the water with a fork and stir. Add honey (or maple and malt syrup mixture) and lemon, and you have in your hands a homemade, herbal sore throat dream.

• **Ginger** – Ginger can be a boon to a sore throat, especially when it occurs with colds or flu. Make a hot tea of fresh root and add lemon—if you're brave, add Garlic. Ginger's pungent heat soothes the inflamed skin, while killing off any viral presence.

• **Mint** – *Menthol* in Mint leaves suppresses cough, and soothes any achy throat. Make a hot tea of it, and perhaps add some lemon or lime. Mint is also mildly anti-viral.

• **Thyme** – Like all these other above herbs, Thyme contains compounds that assuage a sore throat—but also can kill infection-causing microbes that lead up to it. Make a tea of Thyme sprigs with honey (or maple and malt syrup mixture) and lemon. Add crushed Garlic or Ginger if you dare!

Skin Conditions

The health of our skin is important. Not only does it reflect and relay signs about our inner health, it can have a huge impact on our confidence, self-esteem, and appreciation of our looks and beauty.

Of course, while skin conditions aren't always the most painful or life-threatening, they can nonetheless have an enormous impact on how we think and feel. How we portray ourselves to the outside world affects us psychologically. Don't think you look good? This can stress you out—and stress can thus suppress the immune system, leading you closer to illnesses that can and do matter.

Fortunately, herbs—use anciently, and found still in effective products today—have amazing powers of pampering our skin and making us look and feel great. Through my own personal research and practice, the following botanical healers are my choice allies for keeping my skin young and healthy.

Acne

What can be more confidence-crushing than a blemish or blackheads? No matter—these herbal remedies might come in handy, if you're having a bad hair (or skin!) day.

- **Eucalytpus** – A very antibacterial herb, a wash using an infusion or tisane of the dried leaves can cleanse the skin of acne-causing bacteria. Or, add a few essential oil drops to warm water during your morning eau de toilette.

- **Tea Tree** – First-line among topical skin protectors, Tea Tree will decimate acne if used daily. Add a few essential oil drops to warm water for a face wash.

Rash

Dermatitis, allergic reactions, hives, poison ivy, heat rash—no matter the true cause, herbs can help tame your rash within the day. You can trust these following plants especially.

- **Aloe** – For herbalists and even First Aid Kit owners, Aloe leaf gel might be the first go-to for a rash. Apply the gel straight on raised skin, or use Aloe product for any kind of rash—it soothes inflammation and helps with the itching.

- **Plantain** – A salve, oil, or even poulticed leaves can take pain and itching away from rashes of all kinds. Apply Plantain even in cases of poison ivy, oak or sumac, and then rinse it off quickly. You could even prevent a bigger breakout, as Plantain clings to and rinses away rash-causing oils right after touching the plant.

- **Tea Tree** – Use several drops of essential oil, diluted in water, as a wash for poison ivy/sumac/oak **only**. Tea Tree clings to the oils, preventing the rash from spreading. Never apply plain essential oils to bare skin or rashes of other kinds.

Eczema, Dry Skin, and Itch Relief

Eczema sufferers deal with dry, patchy skin, itchiness, and rashes as a chronic auto-immune issue. Since mainstream medications for what is clinically called "atopic" eczema can bring unpleasant side effects, those who deal with it often seek out herbal alternatives.

Others among us may simply have foils with dry skin, flakiness, and itch from time to time. Whether or not you have eczema or just sporadic skin issues, the following herbs are some of the best out there for either.

 • **Aloe** – The inner gel and lotions made from the leaf of this desert plant can relieve dryness, itch, and rash—and speed healing to prevent the further spread of an eczema flare up. Use the plain gel, a salve or oil.

 • **Comfrey** – Moisturizing and pain-relieving, Comfrey might be more adept at helping the skin heal faster after an Eczema flare up than Aloe. Use salve or oil.

 • **Evening Primrose** – Beyond soothing arthritis, Evening Primrose oils—made or bought—can have amazing impact on eczema attacks, as well as itchiness and inflammation. The Omega-3 content assuages the auto-immune issue. Evening Primrose out-performed placebos for eczema outbreaks in many European trials.

Warts

Warts happen. What more, almost all warts are viral in nature—meaning that you could use anti-viral herbs to slow their growth, or remove them completely. It's true that herbs help, but for most wart problems it's best you use mainstream creams, procedures—or talk to your doctor.

• **Garlic** – It will most likely be painful, but crushed garlic has been touted by doctors and herbalists alike for helping shrink warts. You can bandage or tape the crushed clove to your skin for extended periods of time, as well as eat lots of garlic internally.

• **Lemon Balm** – Extracts of this minty, lemony plant have proven highly antiviral. Placing a leaf over the wart, or adding tincture/essential oil directly to warts over time, could speed its removal and shrinkage.

Chapped Lips

Some herbs are moist enough that they can "plump up" and tone the lips. Try making salves out of the following—and yes, you can apply the salve to your chapped lips just like a lip balm, both to further protection and healing.

• **Aloe** – Speeds healing, moisturizes, and helps protect from sun damage to some extent.

• **Comfrey** – Speeds healing and moisturizes.

• **Plantain** – Speeds healing and moisturizes.

Burns

Whether it's from a sunburn, or just an accident in the kitchen, certain plants have been used throughout history to take away burning pains—and to speed healing while reducing scarring. If you experience a minor burn (1st degree) at home, these popular herbs could be excellent first aid.

• **Aloe** – Use of Aloe Vera is practically synonymous with burn healing and relief. Apply the gel or a juice straight to a fresh burn, then rinse of with tepid water after a time. ***Never apply cream, ointment, or salve to an open burn.***

• **Comfrey** – Similar to Aloe, Comfrey achieves the same effects. It cuts down on healing time and even uncomfortable itching. ***Apply in a wash or tea form, but never apply cream, ointment, or salve to an open, unhealed burn.***

• **Plantain** – Itching, healing, pain, and dryness are salved quickly with Plantain. Poultice the plant straight on a burn, or use a tea as a wash—then rinse away in time to let the burn breathe. ***Do not apply salve/cream to unhealed burns.***

• **Rosemary** – This culinary herb comes in handy for skin afflictions. Once a burn is on the way to healing—but you fear lingering infection—a washing tea of Rosemary could calm your fears, and kill residual bacteria.

• **St. John's Wort** – Once the burn is already on its way to healing, apply St. John's Wort to skin that might be itchy or painful. Salve or oil form is best.

• **Tea Tree** – Infected burns could benefit greatly from some Tea Tree. Mix several drops of essential oil in water, and use as a wash or compress if you fear infection. ***Never apply essential oils straight on burns.***

Bug Bites

Mosquitoes, bees, and gnats—oh my! There are sprays and lotions to keep them away. But what about when they have already taken a bite out of your now irritated, stinging skin? Call on these herbs to save the day.

• **Plantain** – In treating bug bites, this is where Plantain truly shines. Chew up some Plantain leaf or seed, and put it straight on your bite. Or, dab a little salve or oil on. Feel the pain and itch go away within minutes.

• **Aloe** – Aloe can help soothe inflamed skin around bug bites in a pinch. Use its plant gel, a bit of juice, or an Aloe Vera ointment or lotion product.

Body Odor

Last but not least—skin can not only make us self-conscious about our looks. If our hygiene gets out of whack, it can also make us very aware of—yes, you guessed it—your personal odor!

Herbs are chock-full of essential, volatile oils, and healing aromas that not only nourish and pamper our skin—they may be able to give us a more pleasant, friendly aroma. Turn to these wonderful-smelling favorites of mine and maybe add them to your cleaning or morning routine!

• **Mint** – A little dash of Mint never hurt anyone. Make a wash using essential oils—add several diluted in water and dab in the areas that count (yes, your pits too).

• **Rosemary** – Rosemary has a nice scent that is neutralizing, stimulating and clarifying. It can also kill peevish bacteria that could be building up stink in your clothes or shoes. Add some essential oils to some water and give yourself a Rosemary bird bath. You'll smell heavenly and invigorating!

• **Tea Tree** – This Australian tree will not only help you mask some unwanted smells, but can also destroy the fungi and bacteria that can raise a funk. A wash made of a few essential oil drops in water can freshen you up—whether it's your body or clothes.

Reproductive or Urinary Maladies

For men and women both, herbs can be our savior—even when dealing with maladies "down under." Before modern pills, ointments or tests, our ancestors and herbalists mastered the use of certain plants for reproductive and urinary issues of all kinds, before they could grow into bigger problems.

Plant medicines that were once depended on for kidney stones, fertility and even child birth are now settled into simpler remedies for minor complications we run into from time to time. Try a few of these out of you run into the stray issue with your menstrual cycle or urinary health.

Menstrual Pain

Got cramps? Stocking up on certain herbs might make you never have to turn to the medicine cabinet again. The following are tried-and-true, studied, and trusted herbs even for the most intense of menstrual pains.

• **Black Haw** – Compounds in the bark and root of this tree mimic the effects of Aspirin. Seek the dried herb, or supplement form, at grocery stores—make the dried bark and roots into a hot tea, taken 2-3 times daily until pains disappear.

• **Black Cohosh** – A tincture or supplement of potent Black

Cohosh can smooth over the pains that come with irregular periods. For the best effect, take a dose twice per day the week before your period. You may enjoy a less painful, heavy feminine symptoms.

• **Ginger** – A powerful anti-inflammatory, Ginger—as food or beverage—taken constantly throughout the day can put any type of cramp at bay. Make a large pot of hot, fresh root tea for the best effect. But you can also eat tons of Ginger in your food, or turn to tinctures and supplements.

• **Lemon Balm** – Calming and cramp-relieving together, Lemon Balm can soothe the smooth muscle of the uterus and really help with PMS. Take a hot tea 3 times per day while you have symptoms, and menstrual pain could hit the road quickly—along with any anxious, unsettled moods you have.

• **Motherwort** – Similar to Lemon Balm, Motherwort can untangle stress or tension related to your period. It can slightly help balance your hormones, and takes away some cramping and bloating that gives you discomfort. Works best in supplement or tincture form, taken 2-3 times per day.

• **Nettles** – Think your cramps are more due to bloating, or water retention? Try infusions of Nettles, or adding the cooked greens to your meals. It's a diuretic—so it will help you rid yourself of excess water weight that leads to menstrual pain.

• **Turmeric** – A pinch of Turmeric powder added to hot water or food can allay your cramping, and your mood. Eat Turmeric-plenty meals all day—or sip infusions at least 3 times a day. Feel the pain go away in time, replaced with warming relief!

U.T.I.'s

These infections always come at the worst times—when we're busy, stressed, or in the midst of combating other health issues.

But herbal allies can help with U.T.I's, before you have to turn to side-effect producing antibiotics. Elect among some of the following urinary-promoting plants that can help cleanse your waterways, remove infection, and get you back to tackling your busy schedule at your best!

• **Garlic** – If you're game for it, do yourself a little "Garlic Cleanse." You can eat anything you want, but you must also chew up or eat crushed Garlic cloves, between 5 and 10 per day! Garlic's antibiotic powers may do just the trick to shorten the duration of your U.T.I.

• **Goldenseal** – You can use Goldenseal topically, internally, or both in the case of a U.T.I. Make a very hot, potent tea from the roots as a wash "down there," or some drops of tincture in water. Take tincture or supplement internally. Goldenseal's berberine can assist your immune system and help destroy the infection itself.

• **Nettles** – Diuretic action can help clear a U.T.I. from your system—and Nettles is your herb. Take Nettle infusions 3 times per day, and drink tons of fluids and water—this could help wash out the infection, with the supporting help of an antibiotic, infection fighting medicine or herb.

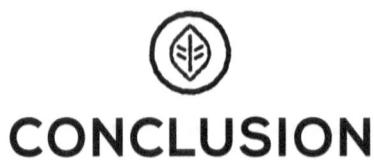

CONCLUSION

Once more, I want to thank you deeply for purchasing *Homemade Herbal Medicine*. If you appreciate the information, or have learned anything fresh and useful in the process, then I feel honored by you—and I consider only one of my many goals as a writer, health-lover, and herb-nerd complete!

Starting out learning herbalism and plant-based home remedies can be difficult, but I hope—and I'm sure—that this book has been an excellent primer for you to continue your journey, get acquainted with the plants, select which ones work best for you—and to empower healing at home.

There is a lot of information on herbs out there. I have done my very best, with all honesty in my research and personal quest for the most tried-and-true herbal remedies. If you are inspired, don't hesitate to find yet more truth and information out there on the subject. The world of herbalism is vast and deep—and the deeper you go, the more safe healing, magic, and miracles you'll find!

Interested in yet more herbalism? Please check out my other publications, chock-full of herbal remedies that champion around specific or common ailments of today. Visit **carmabooks.com** for books that include more specific herbal remedies for inflammation issues, skin care, hormone health, gut health, adrenal fatigue, thyroid support, brain function and so much more.

Remember: always use herbs and supplements in a cautious, informed way. **Knowledge is power, and if you are ever in doubt about the state of your health, never hesitate to contact a professional health practitioner and Master**

Herbalist who can help you with these issues. There is a time to use herbs, and then there is a time to go see the doctor. Know the difference!

I will leave you here, but stay connected and in touch with my *Carma Books* community for more books on holistic, natural, and plant-based health. Reach out again soon for more forthcoming, much-talked-about health titles soon, just like *Homemade Herbal Medicine,* along with plenty of experiences and sharing of tips and knowledge on how to empower healing in your own life—and to get the most mileage out of your health potential!

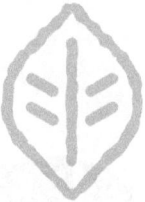

A WORD FROM THE PUBLISHER

Hi, I'm Carmen, a holistic health geek with a passion for health, herbalism, natural remedies, as well as whole-food and plant-based lifestyles. After resolving various health issues I have struggled with for many years, I aim to inspire and help improve your health and longevity by sharing the tireless hours of research and valuable information I have discovered throughout my journey. Through the power of nutrition and lifestyle, with an evidence-based approach, I believe you can achieve your health and wellness goals.

If you enjoyed this book, I would love to hear how it has benefited you and invite you to leave a short review on Amazon - your valuable feedback is always appreciated!

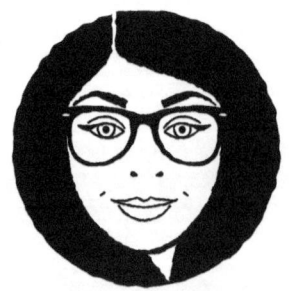

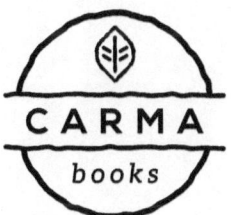

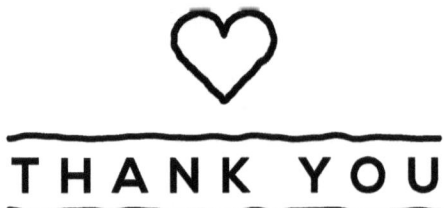

THANK YOU

www.ingramcontent.com/pod-product-compliance
Lightning Source LLC
Chambersburg PA
CBHW050459290526
45786CB00006B/2359